JAN SZAFRAŃSKI

W0006590

Practical Intensive Care Medicine

Acquisitions editor: Melanie Tait
Development editor: Myriam Brearley
Production controller: Chris Jarvis
Desk editor: Jane Campbell
Cover designer: Helen Brockway

Practical Intensive Care Medicine: Problem Solving in the ICU

Charlie Corke MB BS MRCP(UK) FRCA FFICANZCA FANZCA
Director of Intensive Care, The Geelong Hospital,
Victoria, Australia

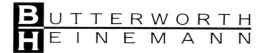

OXFORD AUCKLAND BOSTON JOHANNESBURG MELBOURNE NEW DELHI

Butterworth-Heinemann
Linacre House, Jordan Hill, Oxford OX2 8DP
225 Wildwood Avenue, Woburn, MA 01801-2041
A division of Reed Educational and Professional Publishing Ltd

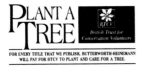 A member of the Reed Elsevier plc group

First published 2000

British Library Cataloguing in Publication Data
Corke, Charlie
    Practical intensive care medicine: problem solving in the ICU
    1. Critical care medicine
    I. Title
    616'.028

Library of Congress Cataloguing in Publication Data
Corke, C. F.
    Practical intensive care medicine : problem solving in the ICU/Charlie Corke.
    p. cm.
    Includes bibliographical references and index.
    ISBN 0 7506 4752 3
    1. Critical care medicine – Examinations, questions, etc. I. Title:
    Problem solving in the ICU. II. Title.
    [DNLM: 1. Intensive Care – Problems and Exercises. WX 18.2 C799p]
    RC86.9 .C67
    616'.028'076–dc21   00–041440

ISBN 0 7506 4752 3

Printed and bound in Great Britain by MPG Books, Bodmin, Cornwall

PLANT A TREE
British Trust for Conservation Volunteers
FOR EVERY TITLE THAT WE PUBLISH, BUTTERWORTH-HEINEMANN
WILL PAY FOR BTCV TO PLANT AND CARE FOR A TREE.

Contents

Introduction

This book is primarily designed to help those junior staff rostered to intensive care, who will immediately find themselves being asked numerous questions concerning the management of unstable patients. You will be expected to come up with correct answers rapidly.

Nursing staff who have worked in intensive care for years, and have usually undergone formal ICU training, will be working out whether or not you are competent, and senior medical staff will not expect to find that you have made incorrect judgements. Most importantly, critically ill patients do not tolerate errors well: your errors are liable to cause significant morbidity and mortality!

Intensive care involves the application of a wide range of medical and physiological knowledge, most of which cannot be acquired by working on the general wards or in the Emergency department. Some appropriate concepts can be learned during an anaesthetic attachment (which is often recommended before working in ICU), but many aspects remain to be grasped.

Ideally, all those working in ICU would receive formal training from experienced ICU staff prior to ever doing a shift as resident on ICU, and would have passed a test to confirm that they have understood all the concepts. While this approach would be ideal, it doesn't happen.

This book is designed to help you to rapidly acquire the knowledge to assist you to work effectively in the intensive care unit. By learning quickly you will become a safe and valuable member of the team, and will get much more from your ICU term than do those who are ill-informed and uncomfortable.

Although you may feel on your own, in reality you are not. Enormous amounts of correct guidance can be obtained from nursing staff and from senior intensive care staff – don't be afraid to ask.

How to use this book

It would be best for you to use this book *before* starting an ICU term. However if you are already working in the area, don't worry: you will benefit by reading it *now*.

Numerous clinical situations are presented in realistic question format. In ICU, data are not presented to you in a vacuum – others have opinions. Sometimes their suggestions will be helpful, but

sometimes they can lead you astray. Both such scenarios are illus-
trated. Read the clinical scenario, then with the answer covered, read
each question carefully and prepare your response before referring to
the answer given.

The straightforward answer to each of the clinical questions is
provided and additional information is included in concise 'mini-
tutorial' format. This format is intended to emulate the bedside
teaching approach.

Where appropriate, for instance those where there is a strong 'evidence base' with a classic paper, references have been included. In
other cases the information presented is based on clinical experience
(e.g. questions on under-water-seal drain or pacing failure), although
this information may be obtained from other books, no specific references are given for these answers.

1

Arterial blood gases

1.1 A 17-year-old girl is admitted to Intensive Care. She is unconscious and ventilated following an overdose of benzodiazepine. Her blood gases are checked on admission to ICU. You are asked if you want to adjust the ventilation.

P_aO_2 (kPa)	pH	P_aCO_2 (kPa)	HCO_3 (mmol/l)	Base excess (BXS) (mmol/l)
13.3	7.60	2.66	19	0

P_aO_2 (mmHg)	pH	P_aCO_2 (mmHg)	HCO_3 (mmol/l)	Base excess (BXS) (mmol/l)
100	7.60	20	19	0

(a) What do the blood gas results show?
The P_aO_2 is normal. The pH reveals an *alkalaemia* – reference to the P_aCO_2 reveals it to be low (normal is 4.66–5.98 kPa or 35–45 mmHg) so there is a *respiratory alkalosis*. The base excess (BXS) is within normal limits (normal +2.5 to −2.5), so there is no metabolic component. This is *acute respiratory alkalosis*.

(b) Do you want to adjust the ventilation?
Yes. The alveolar minute ventilation needs to be reduced – this can be achieved by turning down the tidal volume or reducing the ventilation rate. Usually the rate is reduced. The alveolar partial pressure of CO_2 (P_ACO_2) is directly related to alveolar ventilation: halving the alveolar ventilation will be expected to result in a doubling of the P_aCO_2.

MINI TUTORIAL

P_aO_2 = the partial pressure of oxygen in arterial blood
P_AO_2 = the partial pressure of oxygen in the alveolar gas

F_iO_2 = fractional inspired oxygen concentration. It is an alternative to using percentages to express how much oxygen a patient is receiving:

100% oxygen is F_iO_2 1.0
40% oxygen is F_iO_2 0.4
Room air is F_iO_2 0.21

You need a simple scheme for interpretation of blood gases such as that outlined here:

- Look at the P_aO_2 (and the F_iO_2 where marked).
- Look at the pH and determine acidosis or alkalosis.
- Look at the P_aCO_2 and standard bicarbonate (or base excess) to determine respiratory and metabolic components;

There are a few points which help with interpretation:

- The primary abnormality (respiratory or metabolic) is almost always that which explains the observed pH.
- Compensation is almost always incomplete and only moderates the effect of the primary abnormality.

Both standard bicarbonate and base excess (BXS) are measures of the metabolic status which are uninfluenced by the P_aCO_2 (both are adjusted by the machine to a P_aCO_2 of 5.32 kPa/40 mmHg). The normal range for BXS is +2.5 to −2.5. Positive numbers indicate alkalosis, negative numbers indicate acidosis. The BXS or standard bicarbonate change when metabolic compensation occurs.

1.2 At 2 a.m. the night intern brings an arterial blood sample to ICU from a 71-year-old man who is on the medical ward with a diagnosis of lobar pneumonia. She is worried that he has received too much oxygen (40%) and the F_iO_2 should be reduced.

P_aO_2 (kPa)	pH	P_aCO_2 (kPa)	HCO_3 (mmol/l)	BXS
10.64	7.15	8.64	22	−8

P_aO_2 (mmHg)	pH	P_aCO_2 (mmHg)	HCO_3 (mmol/l)	BXS
80	7.15	65	22	−8

(a) What do the blood gas results show?
The P_aCO_2 is within normal limits (although this requires 40% inspired oxygen to achieve, so the alveolar–arterial gradient is increased). The pH reveals a severe *acidaemia* – reference to the P_aCO_2 reveals a high P_aCO_2 so there is a *respiratory acidosis*. The base excess

(BXS) is low, so there is also *metabolic acidosis*. This is *mixed respiratory and metabolic acidosis.*

(b) What will you tell the intern?
The patient does not have a metabolic alkalosis compensating for chronic CO_2 retention. This is respiratory failure complicated by metabolic acidosis (lactic acidosis due to sepsis in this case). Dropping the F_iO_2 is inappropriate: he is really sick and needs to be reviewed urgently and will probably require ICU admission (unless there are other contraindications).

1.3 Some days later the same intern shows you these arterial blood gas results from a 73-year-old lady who has been admitted to the medical ward with recent onset atrial fibrillation. She has been diagnosed with chronic obstructive airways disease (COAD) and has smoked heavily for more than 50 years. She asks you if these gases are consistent with chronic CO_2 retention.

P_aO_2 (kPa)	pH	P_aCO_2 (kPa)	HCO_3 (mmol/l)	BXS
6.65	7.35	8.512	34	+5

P_aO_2 (mmHg)	pH	P_aCO_2 (mmHg)	HCO_3 (mmol/l)	BXS
50	7.35	64	34	+5

(a) What do the blood gas results show?
The P_aCO_2 is low (we don't know if she is on any supplemental oxygen). The pH reveals a *borderline acidaemia* – reference to the P_aCO_2 reveals a high P_aCO_2 so there is a *respiratory acidosis*. The base excess (BXS) is high, so there is also *metabolic alkalosis*. Since the pH is on the acidotic of 7.4 the acidosis is likely to be the primary abnormality and the metabolic alkalosis is therefore appropriate renal compensation.

(b) Is she right this time?
Yes, this is compensated respiratory acidosis and is entirely consistent with chronic CO_2 retention.
   Hypoxic drive is possibly important for this lady and it is wise to monitor her arterial P_aCO_2 if increased oxygen is administered.

1.4 The medical resident asks you to review a 65-year-old man who is on the surgical ward for management of his peripheral vascular disease. He has become increasingly septic and

appears to be in respiratory distress. The resident has got some arterial blood gas results, but he is uncertain if the gases explain why this man is dyspnoeic.

P_aO_2 (kPa)	pH	P_aCO_2 (kPa)	HCO_3 (mmol/l)	BXS
22.6	7.15	3.32	8.4	−18.6

P_aO_2 (mmHg)	pH	P_aCO_2 (mmHg)	HCO_3 (mmol/l)	BXS
170	7.15	25	8.4	−18.6

(a) What do these results show?
The P_aO_2 is high (he must be on supplemental oxygen). The pH reveals a *marked acidaemia* – there is a low base excess (BXS) so there is a *metabolic acidosis*, reference to the P_aCO_2 reveals a low P_aCO_2 so there is a *respiratory alkalosis*. Since the pH is acidotic the metabolic acidosis is likely to be the primary abnormality and the respiratory alkalosis is compensating. This is therefore partially compensated severe metabolic acidosis.

(b) Do the gases help to explain why the patient is dyspnoeic?
Yes. He is hyperventilating to compensate for a marked metabolic acidosis. Attempts to reduce his ventilation (apart from finding and treating the cause of the acidosis) are inappropriate and detrimental.

1.5 These gases have been brought down from the orthopaedic ward from a patient who the night intern says he is worried about because he is semi-conscious and peripherally shut down. He comments that 'at least the P_aCO_2 is normal'.

P_aO_2 (kPa)	pH	P_aCO_2 (kPa)	HCO_3 (mmol/l)	BXS
5.19	7.16	5.59	14.5	−14

P_aO_2 (mmHg)	pH	P_aCO_2 (mmHg)	HCO_3 (mmol/l)	BXS
39	7.16	42	14.5	−14

(a) Can you summarise the abnormalities for him?
The P_aO_2 is dangerously low. The pH reveals a *marked acidaemia* – there is a low base excess (BXS), so there is a *metabolic acidosis*. Reference to the P_aCO_2 reveals it to be once again within normal limits. Since the pH is acidotic it would be expected that a compensating respiratory alkalosis would be present.

(b) Is there anything you might like to say to him about the P_aCO_2?

The P_aCO_2 is within the normal range, but in the face of the acidaemia a vigorous respiratory compensation (hypocarbia) would be expected. Possible causes of inadequate respiratory compensation include central nervous system depression, respiratory muscle dysfunction or pulmonary pathology.

MINI-TUTORIAL

Patients who may have been hyperventilating to compensate for a metabolic acidosis may be unable to maintain the high minute volume as they become more unwell. Consequently the CO_2 rises, and the pH moves progressively from *compensated metabolic acidosis* to *uncompensated metabolic acidosis* and finally, as the CO_2 rises above normal, to a *mixed acidosis*.

(c) Since you are a little slow getting up to the ward to see the previous patient (due to an unstable patient in ICU) the intern shows you more recent blood gases:

P_aO_2 (kPa)	pH	P_aCO_2 (kPa)	HCO_3 (mmol/l)	BXS
5.45	6.86	6.92	9	−26

P_aO_2 (mmHg)	pH	P_aCO_2 (mmHg)	HCO_3 (mmol/l)	BXS
41	6.86	52	9	−26

Can you summarise the abnormalities for him now?

The P_aO_2 is still dangerously low. The pH reveals a *very severe acidaemia* – there is a low base excess (BXS) so there is a *metabolic acidosis*, reference to the P_aCO_2 reveals that it is now high (*respiratory acidosis*). He has now developed *mixed acidosis*.

(d) What are you going to suggest needs to be done?

This patient still needs urgent review and intervention NOW, before he suffers an arrest. However, it is unlikely you will get to the ward before hearing the code called.

1.6 The night intern mentions a girl to you who is on the ward following an appendicectomy. He says she has been

hyperventilating and he has had her rebreathing from a brown paper bag. He has done some blood gas measurements, which he lets you see.

P_aO_2 (kPa)	pH	P_aCO_2 (kPa)	HCO_3 (mmol/l)	BXS
26.47	7.11	1.86	4.3	−15.8

P_aO_2 (mmHg)	pH	P_aCO_2 (mmHg)	HCO_3 (mmol/l)	BXS
199	7.11	14	4.3	−15.8

Do you have any comment to make?
This girl has a marked *metabolic acidosis* with a compensating *respiratory alkalosis*. Her hyperventilation is an appropriate response to her acidosis; getting her to rebreathe (which raises the P_aCO_2 and can be used to reduce symptoms of acute respiratory alkalosis in hysterical hyperventilation) is utterly inappropriate here. We need to determine why she is so acidotic. Is she shocked (resulting in a lactic acidosis) or is this ketoacidosis? Testing the urine here confirmed ketones: she was an undiagnosed diabetic with ketoacidosis.

1.7 A 73-year-old woman with chronic severe emphysema has worsening of respiratory distress on the surgical ward after a hysterectomy. The following blood gas results are obtained:

P_aO_2 (kPa)	pH	P_aCO_2 (kPa)	HCO_3 (mmol/l)	BXS
8.1	7.43	8.51	41.3	+14

P_aO_2 (mmHg)	pH	P_aCO_2 (mmHg)	HCO_3 (mmol/l)	BXS
61	7.43	64	41.3	+14

The surgical registrar thinks that her high CO_2 indicates that she has respiratory failure, while the medical registrar thinks it is simply a compensation for her metabolic alkalosis.

Who do you think is nearer the truth?
The pH is on the alkalaemic side of normal, suggesting that the metabolic alkalosis is the primary abnormality and the respiratory acidosis is compensatory. However, P_aCO_2 rarely rises above 55 mmHg (7.3 kPa) in respiratory compensation, making the value of 64 mmHg (8.51 kPa) seen here too high simply to be explained by compensation. The surgical registrar is right.

1.8 A surgical patient has had a stormy time in ICU following a colonic anastomotic breakdown. She has been ventilated for two weeks and has a tracheostomy. She is in the process of being weaned. You are asked if you are going to 'do something about the alkalosis'.

P_aO_2 (kPa)	pH	P_aCO_2 (kPa)	HCO_3 (mmol/l)	BXS
11.17	7.44	7.05	35	+10

P_aO_2 (mmHg)	pH	P_aCO_2 (mmHg)	HCO_3 (mmol/l)	BXS
84	7.44	53	35	+10

What are you going to say?
The pH is on the alkalaemic side. There is a *metabolic alkalosis*, but the P_aCO_2 is high (respiratory acidosis), so there is respiratory compensation.

Metabolic alkalosis is common in ICU patients. Correction of the alkalosis may increase respiratory drive and facilitate weaning. Acetazolamide (Diamox) is commonly used to correct metabolic alkalosis. Alternatives are arginine hydrochloride or dilute hydrochloric acid.

1.9 A patient with deteriorating chronic cardiac failure, treated with diuretics, and a recent peptic ulcer, for which he has been taking alkali tablets, becomes unresponsive in the medical ward. The following blood gas results are obtained:

P_aO_2 (kPa)	pH	P_aCO_2 (kPa)	HCO_3 (mmol/l)	BXS
4.52	7.58	6.74	46	+25

P_aO_2 (mmHg)	pH	P_aCO_2 (mmHg)	HCO_3 (mmol/l)	BXS
34	7.58	50.7	46	+25

The medical intern thinks that the high CO_2 is the cause of his conscious state.

What do you think?
No, the hypercarbia is not the cause.

This man is very hypoxic, and this could be the cause of his change in conscious state (other possibilities include cerebral vascular accident (CVA)).

Presumably he is not on supplemental oxygen (if he is, then he is really sick!). He is very alkalaemic with a metabolic alkalosis (high base excess, high bicarbonate). His high CO_2 is compensating for his alkalosis.

He may be a chronic CO_2 retainer (resulting in his high bicarbonate), but at present the metabolic alkalosis is excessive, resulting in an alkalaemia. If his metabolic alkalosis is corrected (with acetazolamide, arginine hydrochloride or hydrochloric acid), then his respiratory drive may increase and his hypoxia improve.

MINI-TUTORIAL

There is a strong reluctance to administer oxygen to patients with CO_2 retention, even when they are very severely hypoxic. These patients can be given sufficient oxygen to improve their oxygenation without undue concern that the CO_2 will rise significantly. Aiming for an oxygen saturation of 90% and a P_aO_2 of 60 mmHg (8 kPa) is appropriate.

These patients require monitoring of their respiratory rate, conscious state and arterial P_aCO_2 when supplemental oxygen is administered.

1.10 You are asked to see a 74-year-old lady who has become unconscious on the medical ward. She has COAD and is known to be a 'CO₂ retainer'. She has been on oxygen, but this was removed after she was found to have become hypercarbic. Your advice is sought to help to decide what to do next.

Time	12.10	13.00	14.50
F_iO_2	0.21	0.4	0.21
PH	7.317	7.305	7.34
P_aCO_2 mmHg (kPa)	71.7 (9.54)	100.3 (13.34)	84.1 (11.18)
P_aO_2	52.7 (7.01)	83.6 (11.12)	23.2 (3.08)
HCO_3	35.5	48.8	44.8
BXS	6.8	10.8	14.4

(a) Can you suggest why this patient might be unconscious?
She is severely hypoxic.

She is likely to be chronically hypoxic anyway; however, the raised P_aCO_2 resulting from the increased oxygen she was given earlier (40%) will be in equilibrium with the alveolar gas (P_ACO_2), and therefore the high CO_2 will be diluting the oxygen in the alveolus – which is only 21% after mask removal (see the explanation of the alveolar gas equation below).

A patient with a high level of CO_2 will effectively get less than 21% oxygen when breathing air, since the oxygen is diluted in the alveolus by the excreted carbon dioxide.

In normal people there is a gradient of 10 mmHg (1.33 kPa) between the alveolar oxygen (P_{AO_2}) and the arterial oxygen (P_{aO_2}).

(b) What will you suggest might help?
She needs oxygen. A small increase may have a useful effect on her P_{aO_2} and conscious level, while not causing the P_{aO_2} to rise unduly. She was given 28% oxygen and became fully conscious in 10 minutes.

MINI-TUTORIAL

The alveolar gas equation is useful to explain the relationship between the inspired oxygen concentration and the arterial $P_{a}CO_2$ with the alveolar oxygen (and consequently the arterial oxygen) partial pressure (P_{aO_2}).

For example (using kPa):

$$P_{AO_2} = F_iO_2 (Pb - P_{H_2O}) - P_{a}CO_2/RQ$$
$$= 0.6(101\text{-}6) - 9.6/0.8$$
$$= 55 - 12$$
$$= 43 \text{ kPa}$$

P_{AO_2} = partial pressure of alveolar oxygen
F_iO_2 = fractional inspired oxygen concentration.
Pb = atmospheric pressure
P_{H_2O} = partial pressure of water vapour
$P_{a}CO_2$ = partial pressure of arterial carbon dioxide
RQ = respiratory quotient

1.11 A 34-year-old man is brought in unconscious having been found in a car with the engine running and a hose from the exhaust through the window. There are also empty benzodiazepine packets and an empty whisky bottle in the car. In the Emergency department the following blood gas results are obtained on 40% oxygen (the saturation is a co-oximeter reading):

P_aO_2 (kPa)	S_aO_2	pH	P_aCO_2 (kPa)	HCO_3 (mmol/l)
4.26	50%	7.38	6.38	28

P_aO_2 (mmHg)	S_aO_2	pH	P_aCO_2 (mmHg)	HCO_3 (mmol/l)
32	50%	7.38	48	28

At the time the blood was taken the transcutaneous pulse oximeter (S_pO_2) was reading 65%. The Emergency registrar says that it is clear that the patient is significantly poisoned with carbon monoxide.

Is he correct?
Yes. The co-oximetry value for oxygen saturation on the blood gas machine is not measuring carboxyhaemoglobin, while the pulse oximeter measures carboxyhaemoglobin as oxyhaemoglobin. Consequently the pulse oximeter reads higher in the presence of carbon monoxide poisoning than does the co-oximeter. The difference in percentage is the percentage of carboxyhaemoglobin. The second clue is that a P_aO_2 of 32 mmHg (4.26 kPa) at a normal pH should give a saturation of about 60%; the low saturation (50%) is due to carbon monoxide.

MINI-TUTORIAL

This patient is very hypoxic (very low P_aO_2). Carbon monoxide alone should not cause this; other causes such as smoke inhalation should be considered. Patients exposed to carbon monoxide need to be on 100% oxygen to optimise oxygen carriage to tissues and to enhance carbon monoxide dissociation. The role of hyperbaric oxygen is controversial.

Scheinkestel CD, Bailey M, Myles PS, Jones K, Cooper DJ, Millar IL, Tuxen DV. Hyperbaric or normobaric oxygen for acute carbon monoxide poisoning: a randomised controlled clinical trial. *Med J Aust.* 1999; **170**(5): 203–10.

2

Respiratory

2.1 An adult patient is admitted ventilated from the ward following resuscitation from a cardiopulmonary arrest. On admission to ICU he is placed on a mechanical ventilator (10 ml/kg tidal volume = 700 ml breaths × 12/min). On admission the peak inspiratory pressure is 40 cm H_2O and the endotracheal tube is at 30 cm (into the trachea from the mouth).

(a) Is a peak inspiratory pressure of 40 cm H_2O in a ventilated patient abnormal?

The normal peak inspiratory pressure in a ventilated patient with normal lungs is usually about 20 cm H_2O. Lower values suggest a leak; higher values suggest obstruction.

(b) Is 30 cm at the mouth a reasonable length for a correctly positioned endotracheal tube?

In adults a correctly positioned endotracheal tube is about 22 cm at the mouth. The tip of a correctly positioned tube should lie opposite the top of the aortic knuckle on CXR. Tubes which are at more than 25 cm at the mouth are almost invariably in the right main bronchus. Nasal tubes are about 4 cm longer at the nostril when correctly positioned.

(c) Is 10 ml/kg a reasonable tidal volume at which to ventilate an ICU patient?

Yes. 10–12 ml per kg or 700–900 ml are appropriate tidal volumes for ventilation in an average adult.

(d) What is the likely problem and how should it be rectified?

The endotracheal tube tip is in the right main bronchus, so all the ventilation is going to the right lung, causing over-distension and higher peak inflation pressures. There is a risk of pneumothorax and of collapse of the unventilated left lung with increased shunt and hypoxia.

The tube should be pulled back to about 22–23 cm.

2.2 Following an increase of a patient's inspired oxygen from 40% to 45%, arterial blood gases are checked to evaluate the response. Oxygen results are:

P_aO_2 80 mmHg
S_aO_2 95%

Is the oxygenation satisfactory or do you want to further increase the oxygen being administered?
No, this is fine. No alteration is required.

MINI-TUTORIAL

The aim with oxygenation is to have an S_aO_2 (arterial oxygen saturation) of between 93 and 95% which corresponds to a P_aO_2 (partial pressure of oxygen) 70–80 mmHg (9.3–10.64 kPa). It would be unusual to accept lower results and would be usual to reduce inspired oxygen (especially when more than 50% oxygen is being administered) when the P_aO_2 is reliably above 90 mmHg (12 kPa).

2.3 You are asked to review an 80-year-old man who is being mechanically ventilated for bronchopneumonia. You are asked if you want to adjust the ventilator settings. Rapid review of his ICU chart reveals the following:

respiratory rate	16
peak inspiratory pressure	27
exhaled tidal volume	70
F_iO_2	0.4 (40%)
pH	7.53
P_aO_2 mmHg (kPa)	53 (7.05)
P_aCO_2 mmHg (kPa)	25 (3.32)

(a) What significant abnormalities are revealed by the blood gas results?
There is a respiratory alkalosis (low P_aCO_2) and hypoxia.

(b) What do you want to do to rectify the situation?
The respiratory alkalosis can be corrected by reducing the alveolar ventilation. This can be achieved by reducing either the tidal volume or the rate. In general, higher than normal tidal volumes (10–12 ml/kg) are used in patients on mechanical ventilation to

avoid atelectasis; consequently, over-ventilation is best tackled by reducing the respiratory rate. Hypoxia is mainly corrected by manipulation of the F_iO_2 (or to a lesser extent by addition of PEEP and increasing mean inspiratory pressure manipulations – see below).

2.4 A 45-year-old man is ventilated in 'Control' mode. He is starting to awake.

What do you anticipate will happen with regard to his ventilation?
He will start to struggle and to fight a ventilator which is set in 'Control' mode.

MINI-TUTORIAL

Controlled ventilation is intermittent positive pressure ventilation (IPPV). A fixed (set) volume is delivered at a fixed rate. No voluntary breaths are possible and attempts are met by no gas (like a hand over the mouth). This readily causes panic in patients, and consequently patients on controlled ventilation require heavy sedation and often paralysis to tolerate it.

Controlled ventilation is now rarely used in ICU, but can be used in paralysed or apnoeic unconscious patients.

2.5 You observe that a patient is in 'Assist Control' mode. The respiratory rate is recorded as 20/minute while the ventilator is set at 12/minute. You are asked to explain what is going on.

(a) What will you say?
This is easily explicable in the Assist Control mode. In assist control the rate will be determined by the number of respiratory efforts that the patient makes (in the absence of patient effort, the rate will be that which is set).

MINI-TUTORIAL

In an Assist Control mode (otherwise termed 'Triggered' ventilation) there is a fixed volume breath delivered at a set rate. Where the patient is making respiratory effort this effort can initiate a mandatory breath. Where the patient attempts to breathe at a higher rate than the mandatory set rate then each effort initiates a breath of the same volume as the mandatory breaths.

Assist Control ventilation is more comfortable for patients than is Controlled ventilation. However, the patient may not be satisfied by the preset volume (the patient may want bigger or smaller breaths). Since every effort results in a relatively large breath, overventilation is common in Assist Control mode.

Assist Control is often used in the USA, but is uncommon elsewhere.

2.6 A patient on Assist Control has a respiratory rate of 45/minute. It is suggested that were you to reduce the sensitivity (making it harder to initiate a breath) this would reduce the rate.

Is this a good idea?

Probably not. If the patient is struggling to breathe (hence the rapid rate), then making it more difficult (reduced sensitivity = harder sucking required to initiate a breath) is not likely to help. However, if the ventilator is triggering itself (auto-cycling) then it is appropriate to adjust the sensitivity to increase the threshold at which a breath is triggered. Auto-cycling is unusual, while respiratory distress or agitation occur more commonly. Observation of the patient (both on and off the ventilator) should suggest the cause of the tachypnoea.

MINI-TUTORIAL

Sometimes, when water precipitates in the ventilator circuit, changes in pressure or flow can result (depending on whether the ventilator is pressure or flow triggered) which the ventilator interprets as a voluntary respiratory effort. This is termed auto-cycling. When auto-cycling the ventilator cycles directly from exhalation to inspiration, and this will occur even when the patient is disconnected and is replaced in the circuit by a bag. Auto-cycling is addressed by removing water from the circuit. Should this fail to rectify the situation it is necessary to adjust the sensitivity.

2.7 The surgical registrar notes that a patient he operated on yesterday is on SIMV ventilation mode. He asks you why the patient is still 'fully ventilated'.

What will you tell him?
The patient may be fully ventilated by a SIMV mode (Synchronised Intermittent Mandatory Ventilation), but may take additional breaths between the set (mechanical) breaths. During weaning the mandatory rate is progressively reduced, and the patient must take more spontaneous breaths.

By looking at the ventilator screen you can determine how many spontaneous breaths the patient is taking and how many mandatory breaths are being given.

MINI-TUTORIAL

In Synchronised Intermittent Mandatory Ventilation (SIMV), there is a preset fixed volume at set rate. The ventilator attempts to deliver these breaths when the patient starts a spontaneous breath (i.e. the breath is synchronised with the patient's inspiration). However, if no respiratory effort occurs within a set interval the breath is delivered anyway. In addition, voluntary efforts to breathe during the time between the set breaths are satisfied by a flow of gas (so between mandatory ventilator breaths patients can take their own breaths, of whatever size they wish).

When the mandatory rate is high, patients do not need to take additional breaths (and be completely mechanically ventilated), but as the mandatory rate is reduced patients take more (spontaneous) breaths on their own. This makes reduction of IMV rate an easy weaning method.

It is important to recognise that patients who are on low rates of SIMV, who are taking most of their minute ventilation spontaneously, will underventilate if given heavy sedation or muscle relaxants (since these will suppress the spontaneous ventilation).

The SIMV mode is very commonly used in ICU.

2.8 Looking at the ventilator you see that a patient is on 15 cm H_2O of Pressure Support. A keen medical student is reviewing the patient and asks what Pressure Support means.

What will you tell him?
Positive pressure is applied whenever the patient takes a spontaneous breath – no breaths occur without patient effort in this mode (although many ventilators have the facility to switch to a backup controlled ventilation should the patient become apnoeic).

MINI-TUTORIAL

Pressure Support can be used to compensate for extra work of breathing due to ventilator inefficiency and resistance caused by endotracheal tubes and connections.

Increasing levels of pressure support will progressively reduce the work the patient needs to do to achieve a given minute ventilation. At 20 cm pressure support a patient with normal lungs would be essentially fully ventilated.

Pressure Support can be used as a sole ventilation mode for those with high work of breathing but good ventilatory drive, or can be used in conjunction with SIMV (usually at a low level of 5–10 cm H_2O) to reduce the additional work associated with spontaneous breaths.

2.9 The student goes on to ask how Pressure Control differs from Pressure Support.

What will you tell him now?
In Pressure Control ventilation a preset pressure is delivered at a fixed (set) rate, while Pressure Support augments spontaneous breaths.

2.10 The student is still really interested and wants to know what advantages Pressure Control offers.

What advantages will you propose?
In Pressure Control the ventilator will generate the set pressure regardless of leaks. Oxygenation may be improved in patients with diffuse lung injury who are ventilated with Pressure Control.

MINI-TUTORIAL

In Pressure Control the ventilator will generate the set pressure regardless of leaks.

Ventilation is better delivered to a patient with a large leak (e.g. big bronchopleural fistula) with Pressure Control ventilation than with standard (volume) controlled ventilation.

Children with uncuffed endotracheal tubes always have a leak (or they should have – lack of leak indicates that the tube is too big and tight in the airway) and are routinely ventilated with Pressure Control.

Pressure in volume control rises progressively as more gas enters the lung; peak pressures occur only at the end of inspiration. In Pressure Control the pressure is constant (at the set inspiratory pressure) throughout the inspiratory phase. Airways with long time constants (i.e. those which inflate slowly during inspiration) are better ventilated when exposed to pressure over a longer period. Oxygenation may improve in patients with severe hypoxia when a Pressure Control mode of ventilation is used.

2.11 A student nurse, new to ICU, says that he is a bit unclear about CPAP (Continuous Positive Airway Pressure) and PEEP (Positive End Expiratory Pressure). He asks you to explain the difference to him.

What will you say?
PEEP is an airway pressure above atmospheric (i.e. positive) at the end of exhalation during mechanical ventilation.

CPAP refers to a positive airway pressure maintained throughout spontaneous breathing.

PEEP maintains functional residual capacity (FRC) and alveolar recruitment in recumbent ventilated patients. Lung water is redistributed from the alveoli to the perivascular interstitial space. Both effects enhance oxygenation.

Maintenance of recruitment reduces lung injury due to shear forces, and increasing FRC may reduce the work of breathing.

CPAP is analogous in spontaneously breathing patients.

2.12 An 82-year-old man is admitted to ICU with fulminant pulmonary oedema. He is tachypnoeic (45/min) and distressed, with sweating and central cyanosis. Non-invasive ventilation is suggested. Is this a reasonable idea? What settings would you suggest?

What will you say?
Yes: this is widely and successfully used in this situation. Starting with 5 cm H_2O expiratory pressure, 10 cm H_2O of Pressure Support and 100% O_2 is reasonable.

MINI-TUTORIAL

Positive expiratory pressure (CPAP or PEEP) is very useful to enhance oxygenation in pulmonary oedema. Work of breathing may also be reduced by increasing FRC in response to PEEP.

The lungs of patients with pulmonary oedema are heavy and non-compliant, which results in an increase of respiratory work. At the same time there is poor oxygen delivery to respiratory muscles as a consequence of desaturation and possibly reduced cardiac output. Pressure support assists inspiration and may be useful. Although CPAP can resolve many cases, the combination of Pressure Support, positive end expiratory pressure and 100% oxygen is probably best. The need for endotracheal intubation has been shown to be reduced by the use of non-invasive ventilation. In addition, ICU stay and complication rates appear to be lower in patients who receive non-invasive ventilation.

Patients with exacerbation of COAD have been shown to benefit from non-invasive ventilation.

In general terms, patients with muscle fatigue and hypercarbia will be most likely to improve with Pressure Support, while those with predominant hypoxia may derive more benefit from CPAP.

Antonelli M, Conti G, Rocco M, Bufi M, De-Blasi RA, Vivino G, Gasparetto A, Meduri GU. A comparison of noninvasive positive-pressure ventilation and conventional mechanical ventilation in patients with acute respiratory failure. *N. Engl. J. Med.* 1998; **339**(7): 429–35.

2.13 You are just phoning the ICU consultant to tell her about an intubated patient you have admitted from the Emergency department. During the conversation she asks you if the endotracheal tube is 'high–low'.

(a) What does she mean?
She wants to know whether the endotracheal tube has *a high volume low pressure* cuff. If it has a standard cuff then it should probably be changed.

(b) Why are these tubes used in ICU?
Since endotracheal intubation is prolonged in patients in intensive care, it is important to avoid damage to tracheal mucosa caused by high pressure from the cuff. High pressure on the mucosa prevents capillary perfusion and results in necrosis. Subsequently, fistula formation or scarring with tracheal stenosis may occur.

Damage is minimised by using an endotracheal tube with a high volume low pressure cuff, which distributes pressure more widely over the tracheal wall and usually requires less pressure in the cuff to seal.

MINI-TUTORIAL

Remember that the pressure inside the cuff does not necessarily reflect the mucosal pressure unless the balloon is big and/or the balloon wall very elastic. A very stiff cuff balloon would require great pressure to inflate it, but would not even touch the tracheal wall when small.

In addition to using endotracheal tubes with high volume low pressure cuffs, the cuff pressure is regularly monitored and adjusted to the minimum pressure that prevents leaks (but not more than 35 cm H_2O, as greater pressures are considered damaging).

To avoid unnecessary tube changing it is helpful to encourage doctors outside ICU (e.g. Emergency department and theatre) who intubate patients, knowing that they will end up in ICU, to select an endotracheal tube with a high volume low pressure cuff.

2.14 You are caring for a 67-year-old man who is ventilated for an aspiration pneumonia. He has a large A-a gradient and requires 70% oxygen and 10 cm H_2O of PEEP. He is ventilated at a tidal volume of 10 ml/kg. The respiratory physician says that he thinks the patient has 'collapse' and that he would benefit from 'sighs'.

Do you agree?
There appears to be progressive collapse of lung units as repeated tidal volumes of the same relatively small size are given. Regular larger breaths may recruit collapsed lung and improve oxygenation. Some ventilators can be set to give regular larger breaths ('sighs'). While this might appear a good idea, it appears that patients become accustomed to the smaller volume and get disturbed when a larger volume is given, without warning, by the ventilator. This causes patients to fight the ventilator and become unsettled. Regular hyper-inflation, supervised by nursing staff or physiotherapists, appears to be better tolerated by patients and is preferred in most units.

2.15 A surgical registrar who has recently rotated to your hospital is visiting a patient upon whom the surgical team have operated. The patient is being ventilated and is intubated with an orotracheal endotracheal tube. The registrar says that 'where he was before' patients in ICU usually had nasotracheal tubes. He

suggests that it is really uncomfortable to have an orotracheal tube and that it is 'very poor practice'.

Do you agree with him?
No. A little knowledge is a dangerous thing: he is slightly correct. Oral tubes are generally a bit more uncomfortable, and patients (particularly younger adults) often require more sedation with an oral tube than with a nasal tube, but there is more to the choice between the two.

MINI-TUTORIAL

	Advantages	Disadvantages
Oral	Larger tube size	Uncomfortable
		Can be obstructed by biting
Nasal	More comfortable	Smaller tube size
	More stable (less movement)	Sinusitis
	Easy to secure	Contraindicated:
		• bleeding diathesis
		• base of skull fracture

Nasal tubes are indicated in children, where stability of the tube is valuable. Young children can push out oral endotracheal tubes with their tongue.

Sinusitis has been shown to be very common in patients with nasal intubation in intensive care.

Meduri GU, Mauldin GL, Wunderink RG *et al.* Causes of fever and pulmonary densities in patients with clinical manifestations of ventilator-associated pneumonia. *Chest* 1994; **106**: 221.

Salord F, Gaussorgues P, Marti-Flich J, Sirodot M, Allimant C, Lyonnet D, Robert D. Nosocomial maxillary sinusitis during mechanical ventilation: a prospective comparison of orotracheal versus nasotracheal route for intubation. *Intensive Care Med.* 1990; **16**: 390–3.

2.16 You are asked to review a 34-year-old woman (60 kg) who is being mechanically ventilated following a massive aspiration of gastric content which occurred during a convulsion. She was admitted two hours ago when she was requiring 50% oxygen but is now on 80%. She is on no PEEP. You are asked if PEEP would be a good idea.

SBP	105
MBP	75
CVP	8
respiratory rate	12
peak inspiratory pressure	27
exhaled tidal volume	620
F_iO_2	0.8
pH	7.38
P_aO_2 mmHg (kPa)	71 (9.44)
P_aCO_2 mmHg (kPa)	38 (5.05)

(a) Do you think PEEP is indicated?
Yes. Patients who are hypoxic and require more than 50% oxygen are usually treated with PEEP (Positive End Expiratory Pressure).

MINI-TUTORIAL

PEEP has various effects, including:

- Increasing low FRC towards normal
- Increased respiratory system compliance (where FRC was previously reduced)
- Prevention of alveolar collapse
- Prevention of small airway closure
- Decreased shunt.

In addition, there is evidence that patients with lung damage have regular localised alveolar collapse and re-expansion with each respiratory cycle. In these cases PEEP prevents this and minimises ongoing injury.

Muscedere JG *et al.* Tidal ventilation at low airway pressures can augment lung injury. *Am J Respir Crit Care Med.* 1994; **149**: 1327–34.

(b) What problems might PEEP cause in this patient?
Reduction of venous return and reduced cardiac output (rarely troublesome below 10 cm PEEP, more problematic if the patient is hypovolaemic).
Pneumothorax.

2.17 While you are reviewing a 45-year-old man (60 kg) who is being mechanically ventilated and is on 10 cm H_2O of PEEP there is some debate about the PEEP level which has been

selected. You are asked how you know that 10 cm is the best level of PEEP to use in this case.

What will you say?
This is a controversial point for which there is no clear answer. How the 'best PEEP' for a particular patient at a specific time in their ICU course should be determined has been a matter of discussion for many years. Simplistically, 'best PEEP' is the PEEP level which achieves the best oxygenation without impairing cardiac output.

MINI-TUTORIAL

The determination of 'best PEEP' is complicated by the absence of a widely accepted monitor which determines the best PEEP level to select.

   Variables which may be used to determine 'best PEEP' include oxygen saturation, oxygen delivery, least intra-pulmonary shunt, best tidal compliance and lowest $ETCO_2$:P_aCO_2 gradient. The pressure–volume curve may be used and PEEP set above the lower inflection point on this curve.

   The variation of required PEEP level with different tidal volumes is confusing and, when improved oxygenation is used as an end point, the fact that a beneficial effect may take an hour or so to occur after a change of PEEP makes monitoring difficult in unstable patients. The situation is made even more complex, since the best level of PEEP may vary for different areas of lung in the same patient (particularly when there is patchy pathology). PEEP which is best for injured portions of lung may be excessive for normal or emphysematous lung.

   The PEEP which results in the best oxygen saturation may cause barotrauma to the lung or reduction in cardiac output. In general, most patients with diffuse lung injury (failure of F_iO_2 of 0.5 to maintain an arterial saturation of > 90%) will be considered to have an indication for PEEP.

2.18 You are called to urgently review a 32-year-old man because he has become bradycardic. He is ventilated for ARDS (Acute Respiratory Distress Syndrome) with an SIMV rate of 20/minute, tidal volume of 600 ml and pressure limit of 40 cm H$_2$O. He is on sedation and muscle paralysis. Rapid review of his ICU chart reveals the following:

Time	0700	0720
Heart rate	90	45
Systolic BP	110	60
Respiratory rate	20	20
Peak inspiratory pressure	35	15
Exhaled tidal volume	600	220
F_iO_2	1.0	1.0
P_aO_2 mmHg (kPa)	70 (9.31)	50 (6.65)
P_aCO_2 mmHg (kPa)	45 (5.98)	52 (6.92)

(a) Why has the tidal volume dropped?

The expiratory tidal volume has fallen from 600 to 220 ml and the peak inspiratory pressure, which was high at 35 cm H_2O, is now only 15 cm H_2O. There must be a loss of gas from the circuit. Low exhaled minute volume alarms and low peak pressure alarms on ventilators are designed to detect this serious complication.

(b) Is turning up the tidal volume likely to resolve the situation?

There is a remote chance that it might help in the short term, but this misses the point entirely. The source of the leak must be found and rectified.

(c) What is the most likely cause of this situation?

Leaks usually occur from disconnected tubing (most commonly at the humidifier or endotracheal tube connection). Cuff leakage is less common.

2.19 A 60-year-old woman is ventilated for pneumonia with an SIMV rate of 12 breaths/minute, a set tidal volume of 700 ml and 5 cm of PEEP. The pressure limit is set at 35 cm H_2O. At 1.30 a.m. you are asked to review her because she is sweating and 'fighting' the ventilator and the high pressure alarm keeps going off. An extract from her chart is shown below:

Time	0030	0100	0130
Heart rate	90	130	149
Systolic BP	120	80	60
Respiratory rate	12	24	16
Peak inspiratory pressure	24	30	35
Exhaled tidal volume	700	700	300
F_iO_2	0.4	0.4	0.6
P_aO_2 mmHg (kPa)	100 (13.3)	50 (6.65)	54 (7.18)
P_aCO_2 mmHg (kPa)	42 (5.59)	49 (6.52)	60 (7.98)

(a) What should be done straight away (while you are thinking about the problem)?
This patient is not ventilating well and is hypoxic. The mechanical ventilator may be faulty and it is important to remove patients from the ventilator and manually ventilate them with 100% oxygen when problems occur. Bagging may also give a 'feel' of the tightness of the patient being ventilated.

(b) Why has the exhaled tidal volume gone down?
The increased peak pressure has exceeded the pressure limit. When the pressure exceeds the set pressure limit the ventilator cycles to exhalation, so the patient gets less tidal volume than is set – often very little. In this case the exhaled volume is only 300 ml although the ventilator is set to deliver 700 ml. All the other features result from hypoventilation.

(c) It is suggested that increasing the sedation might help, do you agree?
Patients who are underventilated and/or hypoxic and are dying tend to fight – NEVER explain high pressures as due to 'fighting' until all other causes are excluded with certainty.

(d) What are the most likely causes of this problem and how would you identify each?

Causes of obstruction	Suggested by
Tube blockage (biting or sputum plug)	Passage of suction catheter blocked in tube
Right main bronchial intubation	Checking tube length at mouth, auscultation – silent left side
Sputum plug in main bronchus	Auscultation, tracheal deviation towards silent side, CXR
Pneumothorax	Auscultation, tracheal deviation away from silent side, hyper-resonance, CXR

MINI-TUTORIAL

Exceeding the set pressure limit causes the ventilator to stop pushing in gas and cycle to exhalation.

If the pressure limit is exceeded just at the end of a breath then a reasonable volume breath may have been given, but usually the pressure rockets up and the alarm goes off. In this situation minimal ventilation is being delivered and it is essential the patient is manually bagged to ensure adequate ventilation while the cause of the problem is sought.

2.20 A patient in intensive care with acute pancreatitis has bilateral, predominantly basal, infiltrates on his chest X-ray. On mechanical ventilation, 10 cm of PEEP and 90% oxygen he has a P_aO_2 of 75 mmHg (9.98 kPa). The pulmonary wedge pressure is 12 mmHg. An intern asks you whether you think this patient has ARDS.

What will you say?
There are defined criteria for Acute Respiratory Distress Syndrome (ARDS). This patient satisfies the criteria.

MINI-TUTORIAL

The diagnosis ARDS can be applied to a wide spectrum of lung injury (from bi-basal infiltrates to diffuse pulmonary involvement) due to a myriad of local and systemic causes including:

- Sepsis
- Aspiration
- Primary pneumonia
- Multiple trauma

- Multiple transfusions
- Cardiopulmonary bypass
- Fat embolism
- Pancreatitis.

The criteria for diagnosis have been developed with the main aim of facilitating categorisation of patients with lung disease for research purposes. The American–European Consensus Conference on ARDS arrived at the following definition for ARDS in 1994:

- Acute onset
- P_aO_2/F_iO_2 < 200 mmHg (26.6 kPa)
- Bilateral infiltrates on chest X-ray
- No clinical evidence of high left atrial pressure (PAWP < 18 if measured).

The criteria for acute lung injury (ALI) are similar, but the requirement for decreased oxygenation is less stringent, P_aO_2/F_iO_2 < 300 mmHg (39.9 kPa).

The original description of ARDS included dyspnoea, cyanosis refractory to oxygen, reduced lung compliance and diffuse (rather than simply bilateral) infiltrates on the chest X-ray.

Bernard GR *et al.* The American-European Consensus Conference on ARDS. Definitions, mechanisms, relevant outcomes, and clinical trial coordination. *Am. J. Respir. Crit. Care Med.* 1994; **149**(3 Pt 1): 818–24.

2.21　You are asked to review a 46-year-old woman who is ventilated for ARDS (secondary to an intra-abdominal abscess which has now been drained). She is on SIMV with a rate of 20 breaths/minute, a set tidal volume of 500 ml and 15 cm of PEEP. The pressure limit is set at 35 cm H_2O. She has had routine arterial blood gases performed which are as follows:

F_iO_2	0.9
pH	7.35
P_aO_2 mmHg (kPa)	76 (10.11)
P_aCO_2 mmHg (kPa)	97 (12.90)

The surgeon who performed the laparotomy is at the bedside and is most concerned that the CO_2 is so high. He asks you why the patient isn't being ventilated properly.

What will you say?
It has become accepted practice to limit tidal volume and ventilation pressure in patients with ARDS (to avoid further lung injury) and to

accept the consequent high arterial $P_a CO_2$ levels (this is referred to as 'permissive hypercapnia').

MINI-TUTORIAL

The concept of permissive hypercapnia is that in patients with pulmonary injury who require mechanical ventilation the ventilation is delivered in such a way that further pulmonary injury is prevented or minimised. Damage limitation is achieved by reducing alveolar ventilation, and consequently hypercapnia results. The strategy rests on the observation that hypercapnia has fewer and less significant adverse effects than does ventilation designed to achieve normal $P_a CO_2$ levels in these patients with diseased lungs.

Although there is controversy relating to the strategy of ventilation which is most likely to prevent or minimize lung injury (particularly with respect to PEEP levels), it does seem generally accepted that big swings between inspiratory and expiratory pressures resulting from relatively high tidal volume (> 10 ml/kg) and low PEEP (< 10 cm H_2O) are damaging.

Currently used tidal volumes of 5–7 ml/kg (aiming to keep plateau pressures below 35 cm H_2O) with respiratory rates of < 25/min in patients with ARDS will often result in hypercarbia. The hypercarbia stimulates respiratory drive, but providing the patient is well sedated or paralysed the hypercapnia is generally well tolerated (high CO_2 in the absence of hypoxia does not seem to have significant clinical effects).

A decline in mortality has been suggested by retrospective studies and some prospective studies using this technique.

Amato MB *et al.* Beneficial effects of the 'open lung approach' with low distending pressures in Acute Respiratory Distress Syndrome. A prospective randomised study. *Am. J. Respir. Crit. Care Med.* 1995; **152**: 1835–46.
Hickling KG *et al.* Low mortality rate in adult respiratory distress syndrome using low-volume, pressure limited ventilation with permissive hypercapnia: a prospective study. *Crit. Care Med.* 1994; **22**: 1568–78.

2.22 You are managing a 42-year-old man who has ARDS following meningococcal septicaemia. He has a $P_a O_2$ of 52 mmHg (6.92 kPa) on 100% oxygen. Pneumothorax is excluded and the suggestion is made that he be turned prone (face down). The medical registrar says that he thinks this is a silly idea, which is not likely to be of benefit and will probably result in extubation and emergency intubation.

Is he right?

No. Oxygenation improves in most patients with ARDS when they are turned into the prone position (improvement is often substantial).

Where care is taken during turning removal of lines and tubes should not occur.

MINI-TUTORIAL

The effect of prone positioning on oxygenation has been observed in 32 patients with severe acute respiratory failure (Chatte, 1997). After 1 h in the prone position the P_aO_2 increased by 50%, and 1 h after returning to a supine position there was still an increase of 20% in the P_aO_2 compared with the value before turning.

One in five patients show no improvement. However, those who do respond tend to have repeated improvements in P_aO_2 with subsequent turns into the prone position.

Chatte G *et al.* Prone position in mechanically ventilated patients with severe acute respiratory failure. *Am. J. Respir. Crit. Care Med.* 1997; **155**(2): 473–8.

2.23   A 73-year-old man remains ventilated with a diffuse pulmonary infiltrate after one week of intensive care. He had severe sepsis from an obstructed infected right kidney when he was admitted, but after nephrostomy drainage this has resolved. He now appears to have ARDS and his intra-pulmonary shunt and chest X-ray appearances have remained unchanged for 3 days. The value of lung biopsy and the role of corticosteroids are raised.

What do you think?

Open lung biopsy has low morbidity (particularly when performed by thoracoscopy or mini-thoracotomy) and can be very useful to exclude specific causes of lung infiltrate (including nosocomial infection, tuberculosis, malignancy, vasculitis and bronchiolitis obliterans organising pneumonia (BOOP)). Lung histology may also help to identify patients who are likely to benefit from steroid treatment. Steroids might be helpful in the late fibrotic stage of ARDS, although this remains unresolved.

MINI-TUTORIAL

Pulmonary fibroproliferation (PFP) occurs as a late change in patients with ARDS. Although there are no good prospective studies, there are reports that corticosteroid treatment can assist the resolution of this fibrotic change.

There are histologic features on the open lung biopsy which suggest that there will be a favourable response to steroids. These include preserved alveolar architecture, myxoid type fibrosis and coexistent intraluminal bronchiolar fibrosis. In contrast, the presence of arteriolar subintimal fibroproliferation might suggest that steroids will not be effective.

Meduri G *et al.* Corticosteroid rescue treatment of progressive fibroproliferation in late ARDS. Patterns of response and predictors of outcome. *Chest* 1994; **105**(5): 1516–27.

Meduri G. Levels of evidence for the pharmacologic effectiveness of prolonged methylprednisolone treatment in unresolving ARDS. *Chest* 1999; **116** (1 Suppl): 116S–118S.

2.24 A 70 kg 24-year-old patient is admitted to the ICU from the Emergency department. He has been intubated and ventilated as a result of severe asthma. On admission to ICU he is on the following ventilator settings:

Tidal volume	1000 ml
Rate	16
Inspiratory flow rate	30 l/min
PEEP	5 cm H_2O
Peak pressure limit	35

You are asked to review the settings for continuing ventilation in ICU.

What settings do you suggest and why?
700 ml tidal volume, a rate of 6/min and an inspiratory flow rate of 80 l/min.
   PEEP is generally of no help in asthma.

MINI-TUTORIAL

Gas trapping is now recognised to be a major risk in the ventilated asthmatic. Using high pressures it is possible to get air into almost any lung. However, the pressure driving exhalation will be much lower and flow during exhalation will be slow in the face of significant bronchospasm. Unless adequate time is permitted for exhalation alveoli will 'blow up and explode'. Expiratory time is lengthened by reducing the respiratory frequency or decreasing the inspiratory time (by increasing the inspiratory flow rate) or a combination of the two.

Rapid inspiratory flows (80–100 l/min) and lowish respiratory rates (6–10 /min) are used in ventilated asthmatics in order to maximise expiratory time and reduce the chances of gas trapping. Tidal volumes appear less important, but it would be unusual to choose tidal volumes above 10 ml/kg.

2.25 You come on duty for a night shift and at handover see a 15-year-old girl with asthma who is being ventilated. She is quite stable, but 30 minutes later you are called urgently because she has desaturated (S_pO_2 67%) and become hypotensive (56/32).

What are the most likely causes for this situation?

The most likely cause is over inflation of the lung due to gas trapping. This can result in high pressure in the thorax, causing obstruction to venous return or lung rupture and tension pneumothorax (which also results in obstruction to venous return). The latter is the more likely cause.

MINI-TUTORIAL

Collection of exhaled gas during a prolonged apnoea is presently the best method of measuring gas trapping. VEI (end-inspiratory lung volume) is determined by measuring expiratory volume during a pause in ventilation (i.e. both the tidal volume and trapped gas). The VEI should be kept below 20 ml/kg. (Note: 10 ml/kg is an average tidal volume.)

NB: Waveforms give an idea only, as the machine uses a pneumotachograph to measure expiratory flow. Pneumotachographs may not register the very low expiratory flows in severe asthma. Devices which occlude the airway at the end of the exhalatory period and measure any pressure development may also be used to estimate gas trapping.

Disconnecting the patient from ventilation and establishing that there is a long wheeze (by putting your ear to the tube) as the lung deflates is the simplest method and is therapeutic, since the lung deflates during testing. Intermittent temporary disconnection is important in asthmatics who develop hypotension in ICU or in asthmatics who arrest and are intubated.

Although peak inspiratory pressures (PIP) (as measured at the mouth) rise when high inspiratory flows are used (to maximise expiratory time) the high bronchial resistance prevents this pressure being transmitted to the alveoli (presuming bronchospam is uniform), this may be true in asthma but obstruction in an exacerbation of obstructive airways disease is heterogeneous. Consequently, the risk of alveolar rupture and pneumothorax is not directly related to mouth peak pressures in patients with severe asthma.

2.26 A 22-year-old female, a known asthmatic, has a cardio-respiratory arrest secondary to asthma shortly after arrival in the Emergency department. She is intubated and manually ventilated on 100% oxygen by the anaesthetic registrar, who states he is having difficulty ventilating her. He is using two hands on the bag and is achieving a rate of 15/minute. She has had four doses of intravenous adrenaline and is in electro-mechanical dissociation. The Emergency registrar asks if you have any suggestions.

What will you suggest?
Stop ventilating her and disconnect the bag. She is likely to have massive gas trapping, causing tamponade. The registrar should stop ventilating for a minute and listen to the tube till the wheeze stops. Thinking about exhalation is important. A ventilation rate of 6/minute is probably adequate in severe asthma; giving 100% oxygen maximises oxygenation and reduces the severity of hypoxia during disconnections.

2.27 A 45-year-old woman was admitted to ICU yesterday with an exacerbation of asthma. She needed to be intubated overnight but has improved following treatment with intravenous salbutamol, intravenous steroid and aminophylline. She was extubated 2 hours ago. The salbutamol infusion has ceased. You are called because the lactate is very high. The results are shown below:

pH	7.24
P_aO_2 mmHg (kPa)	98 (13.03)
P_aCO_2 mmHg (kPa)	32 (4.26)
HCO_3	18
lactate	7.2

(a) Why has she got such a lactic acidosis?
Lactic acidosis is common in patients who have been treated with salbutamol (particularly intravenous salbutamol). It is thought that salbutamol may uncouple oxidative phosphorylation, resulting in the acidosis.

(b) What investigations are indicated?
None (other than clinical examination to confirm the absence of shock).

(c) What are you going to suggest to do about it?

While disturbing (to medical staff), this acidosis clears spontaneously. When clinically possible, reduction of intravenous salbutamol administration may facilitate resolution of the lactate level. In patients who continue to have severe bronchospasm, continuation of salbutamol has been shown still to be associated with resolution of the acidosis; consequently continued monitoring may be all that is required.

2.28 You are urgently called to the thoracic surgical ward by a junior nurse who is worried about the massive bubbling occurring in bottle C of an underwater drainage system (Fig. 2.1) connected to a patient who underwent a right upper lobectomy yesterday. He is concerned that increased bubbling indicates that the patient has a bronchopleural fistula.

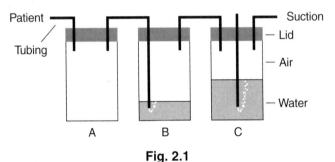

Fig. 2.1

(a) Do you agree?

No. The third bottle (C) is designed to bubble continuously. The wall suction is turned up until bubbling occurs. The amount of suction delivered is adjusted by altering the depth of water in the bottle (if the tube tip is 10 cm under water then suction is 10 cm H_2O below atmospheric pressure). The wall suction may be turned down until the bubbling is gentle but constant.

If bottle B bubbled constantly and furiously it would suggest that the patient had a broncho-pleural fistula.

(b) Can you simply explain the function of each bottle?

A   collects any fluid draining from the chest.

B   a one-way valve (air can leave the patient but not return into the chest) is created in bottle B when the water level is above the bottom of the inlet tube (bubbling here *does* indicate air coming from the chest. (Note: When suction is applied and there is a leak at the joint between the chest tube and tube to the under-water seal, there will also be bubbling in bottle B.)

C   is a system to deliver a determined amount of suction.

(c) What can happen if the suction is turned off but the tubing to the suction is left connected?

Any air leaving the chest cannot get out of the bottles and pressure will build up. This can cause tension in the chest, rapidly in the case of massive air leaks. The disposable underwater drain systems have a relief valve to avoid this possibility, but the suction tubing should always be disconnected from the disposable underwater drain when the suction is turned off.

(d) What is likely to happen if the chest drain is removed or clamped when there is ongoing brisk bubbling in bottle B?

Pneumothorax is likely to occur rapidly and will probably cause intra-pleural tension (tension pneumothorax).

2.29 A 78-year-old man who weighs 65 kg is in the process of being weaned from mechanical ventilation 24 hours following coronary artery grafting. He is breathing on 50% oxygen, 10 cm of CPAP and has 15 cm of Pressure Support. He currently has a respiratory rate of 35 and tidal volume of 420 ml, and he can increase this to 650 ml on request to breath as deeply as he can. The cardiac surgeon tells you he wants him extubated now.

What can you say?

Take the surgeon's request as a suggestion and relay it to your regis-trar or to the ICU consultant. *Do not do it.* This patient is not ready for extubation and will have a very high probability of re-intubation if extubated.

MINI-TUTORIAL

Although a number of parameters have been suggested to predict weaning failure, none stands alone. Features suggesting failure include:

Respiratory rate > 30
Tidal volume < 10 ml/kg
Vital capacity < 1000 ml
Need for pressure support > 10

Need for > 50% oxygen
Rising PAP on weaning
Rising PCWP on weaning.

Increasing respiratory rate with a progressive decrease in tidal volume over time is also a poor feature.

Paradoxical ventilation ('rocking' respiratory pattern where the chest appears to move in as the abdomen moves out), sweating, tachycardia and rising arterial P_aCO_2 are other pointers to impending weaning failure.

The relationship of tidal volume and respiratory rate has been suggested to be a useful predictor of weaning failure. Patients with rapid shallow breathing are predicted to fail:

$f/Vt < 80$ = weaning probable
    (f = respiratory rate, Vt = tidal volume in litres)
$f/Vt > 105$ = weaning failure likely.

The ratio more reliably identifies patients who will fail to wean than those who will succeed.

Yang KL, Tobin MJ. A prospective study of indexes predicting the outcome of trials of weaning from mechanical ventilation. *N. Engl. J. Med.* 1991; **324**(21), 1445–50.

2.30 A 56-year-old woman with an exacerbation of COAD has required ventilatory support. She is currently on CPAP mode with 5 cm of expiratory pressure and 25 cm of pressure support. She has a respiratory rate of 15/minute and is well saturated on 30% oxygen. The medical registrar asks why the patient is not yet extubated.

What will you tell him?

She is still on substantial Pressure Support and is not ready to extubate.

Patients requiring 25 cm of Pressure Support are effectively being fully ventilated (although they are determining the respiratory rate). It is traditional to consider a patient breathing on CPAP as being near extubation. However, with the introduction of Pressure Support it is common to have patients on a CPAP mode on the ventilator while their ventilation continues to be significantly augmented by high levels of Pressure Support. Patients are generally not ready to be weaned while on more than 10 cm of Pressure Support.

2.31 A ventilated man with COAD is recorded to have an auto-PEEP of 12 cm H$_2$O. A medical student says he has heard of PEEP but asks you to explain auto-PEEP to him.

(a) What will you say?
Auto-PEEP (otherwise termed 'intrinsic PEEP') occurs when the ventilator cycles to inhalation before exhalation has finished (this is the same as the trapping concept for asthma already discussed; auto-PEEP can be used as a method of determining the degree of trapping in asthma).

(b) What are its effects?
Auto-PEEP results in increased intra-thoracic pressure which reduces true cardiac filling pressures and confounds pulmonary artery wedge pressure interpretation.

Since auto-PEEP must be reversed before inspiratory airflow can be initiated (and the ventilator triggered) respiratory workload can be high in patients spontaneously breathing (with or without mechanical support).

(c) What will you suggest needs to be done?
Auto-PEEP is reduced by reducing expiratory flow resistance (pharmacologically) or by increasing expiratory time.

2.32 You are caring for a 34-year-old woman with very severe ARDS who is being paralysed to facilitate her ventilation. She is on a pancuronium infusion at 4 mg/h and has been on this dose for 24 hours. It is suggested that she is receiving an excessively large dose neuromuscular blocker.

What do you think? How can you tell?
It is impossible to know without either stopping the infusion and observing her reactions or by testing with 'Train-of-Four' nerve stimulation.

MINI-TUTORIAL

Few patients require prolonged neuromuscular blockade in intensive care, but this is occasionally required in cases of severe asthma or ARDS.

It is important to avoid excessive administration of neuromuscular blocking drug.

When intermittent boluses of neuromuscular blocking drugs are administered it is important to ensure that there is some evidence of recovery of muscle activity between doses. Similarly, continuous infusions should be regularly ceased and restarted only after there is evidence of muscle activity (reduction of dose is appropriate where there is a prolonged period before muscle activity returns).

Additional benefits of regularly lifting neuromuscular blockade include the ability to assess the adequacy of concomitant sedation and analgesia, and to determine the need for continued paralysis.

Peripheral nerve stimulation ('Train-of-Four') is recommended to guide sustained neuromuscular blockade in the ICU.

2.33 It has become evident that a patient in the intensive care unit requires intubation as a result of progressive respiratory failure. Senior assistance is on the way and you are asked to quickly get 'set up' for the intubation.

What will you need to do and what should you obtain?
- The patient (if conscious) needs to be informed of what is being planned, and so do relatives (except in extreme emergency).
- The bed head needs removal and the bed moved out and the head's area cleared to enable easy access for the intubating doctor.
- Suction needs to be checked, connected to a rigid sucker and placed where it can be easily accessed (under the pillow will do well).
- Two functioning (checked) laryngoscopes are required (in case one fails).
- An endotracheal tube of appropriate size – e.g. 8.5 for a man and 8 for a woman (high volume low pressure cuff) with checked cuff (and a second tube of half a size smaller unopened but available).
- Syringe for cuff inflation.
- An intubating stylet (available in case of difficulty).
- A Guedel airway (available in case of difficulty necessitating bag-and-mask ventilation).
- A manual resuscitation bag.
- Materials to secure tube.
- Anaesthetic agents and relaxant drugs.
- Pulse oximetry and an end-tidal CO_2 monitor are recommended.

MINI-TUTORIAL

Anticipate that the effect of the anaesthetic drugs and short-acting relaxant will wear off rapidly after intubation and the patient will start to cough and struggle (particularly if the patient is young and conscious prior to intubation). Anticipate this and have appropriate drugs prepared before intubation, either to give as bolus or as infusion after intubation.

2.34 You have just intubated a 78-year-old man. He requires ventilation due to respiratory failure which is complicating right lower lobe pneumonia. Before intubation his blood pressure was 125/80, but it is now 55/30.

The low pressure is pointed out to you. What do you want to do about it?
Give a bolus of intravenous fluid rapidly (e.g. 500 ml N/saline or 200 ml Haemaccel – and repeat if unresponsive). If this is not rapidly effective give metaraminol 1 mg iv (and repeat as required). If the hypotension is not rapidly corrected then bradycardia and cardiac arrest may develop in very sick patients. (The scenario of endotracheal intubation followed within minutes by arrest is not uncommon).

Consider the possibility that the mechanical ventilation is resulting in gas trapping and that this is causing tamponade and hypotension.

MINI-TUTORIAL

There are a number of factors contributing to the hypotension which predictably occurs after induction and ventilation of severely ill patients:

- Prior to induction, severely ill patients may be very stressed, with high sympathetic drive. This drive will be suddenly reduced following induction of anaesthesia.
- Anaesthetic induction agents (thiopentone, propofol, opiates) have a vasodilating effect.
- Increased mean intra-thoracic pressure resulting from intermittent positive pressure ventilation will reduce cardiac output disproportionately in patients with hypovolaemia and low filling pressures (usual in sepsis).

There are a number of things which can be done to avoid or minimise post-induction hypotension:

- Use minimal doses of induction agent. Some patients are unresponsive before you start and require minimal or no induction agent – in this situation the price of underdosing (possible awareness) is much less than the price of overdosing (death).
- Give a fluid load just before induction when the patient is hypovolaemic, particularly where they are hypovolaemic and peripherally vasoconstricted (because they will inevitably dilate on induction).

2.35 You are caring for a 75-year-old man who is intubated and ventilated for a diffuse pulmonary infiltrate of unknown aetiology. He is undergoing a fibre optic bronchoscopy which is being performed by the respiratory registrar. While the bronchoscopy is being performed the over pressure alarm on the ventilator goes off (checking the ventilator shows it to be set on 40 cm H_2O). The registrar becomes agitated because he thinks he has caused a pneumothorax. He asks you what you think.

What do you think is happening?
The 'high peak pressure' alarm on the ventilator is probably going off because it has not been increased for the procedure and the endotracheal tube is being partially obstructed by the bronchoscope.

MINI-TUTORIAL

The bronchoscope is filling the endotracheal tube lumen and increasing the resistance in the tube.

This is particularly the case with a small endotracheal tube and a big bronchoscope. The pressure in the ventilator circuit (where peak inspiratory pressure is measured) is increased but the high peak inspiratory pressure is not getting to the lung because of the high resistance caused by the scope in the endotracheal tube.

It is appropriate (and necessary) to increase the high-pressure limit during fibre optic bronchoscopy in intubated patients. The chest should be observed for rise to confirm inflation and fall to indicate that trapping is not excessive. Oxygen should be set to 100% for the procedure. A specific endotracheal connector is required through which the bronchoscope can pass (with an airtight seal) while ventilation continues.

Pneumothorax is a risk, particularly where significant trapping occurs due to expiratory obstruction (due to the bronchoscope) and inadequate expiratory time.

It is important to return peak airway pressure settings to the pre-bronchoscopy values after completion of the procedure.

Also expect the low tidal volume or circuit leak alarm to activate during bronchoscopic suctioning, since the tidal volume will be sucked up the bronchoscope and not return to the ventilator to be registered as exhaled tidal volume.

2.36 You are caring for a 56-year-old woman who has been ventilated for 10 days due to a severe exacerbation of COAD. She has had a tracheostomy and weaning from ventilation is proving difficult. On the ward round there is a discussion about weaning and you are asked to outline the factors involved in weaning.

What will you say?
Most simplistically, successful weaning depends upon a favourable balance of respiratory muscle power in relation to required respiratory muscle work.

MINI-TUTORIAL

Consideration of weaning requires:

Minimisation of respiratory work:

Minimum resistance	largest safe endotracheal tube diameter
	shortest safe tube length
	treat bronchospasm
	treat pulmonary oedema
	minimise ventilator machine work
Maximum compliance	treat infection
	treat atelectasis/consolidation
	treat pulmonary oedema
Minimise rebreathing	minimise circuit dead space
Minimise CO_2 production	avoid pyrexia
	avoid struggling/agitation
	avoid over-feeding? substitute fat (no?)
Position	sit up (avoids pushing down abdominal contents and pushing up both abdominal fat and breasts with each breath). When sitting up weight of bowels, abdominal fat and dependent breasts assist inspiration.

Maximisation of respiratory power:

Preserve muscle	feed early
	avoid prolonged muscle paralysis
	continue some respiratory muscle activity where possible with IPPV
	minimise catabolic steroid use
Optimise muscle power	normalise electrolytes (esp. PO_4^{--}, K^+, Ca^{++})
	normalise FRC (CPAP if low, reduce trapping if high)
	maintain cardiac output (where compromised)
	aminophylline
	avoid fatigue (once muscle is fatigued it takes extended time to recover so avoid overdoing weaning periods)
Optimise drive	sedated patients do not generate maximal power so avoidance of long-acting sedatives is desirable

2.37 A ventilated patient has a heat and moisture exchanger (HME) in the inspiratory limb of the ventilator circuit (just before the 'Y' connection). You are asked to explain how it will humidify the gas delivered to the patient.

What will you say?
It won't. A heat and moisture exchanger (HME) works by condensing moisture from exhaled gas and returning this moisture to the dry gas in the next breath. It will only function if both expiratory and inspiratory gas passes through it (it must therefore be positioned between the 'Y' piece in the circuit and the endotracheal tube).

MINI-TUTORIAL

When the upper airway is bypassed by endotracheal intubation (or tracheostomy) during mechanical ventilation it is essential that the ventilation gases be humidified to avoid drying of sputum, with consequent airway plugging. Humidification can be accomplished using either a heated humidifier or a heat and moisture exchanger (HME).

Heated humidifiers result in active humidification and increase the heat and water vapour content of inspired gas. HMEs are passive humidifiers and store heat and moisture from the patient's exhaled gas and then release it to the inhaled gas in the next breath. Humidifiers should provide a minimum of 30 mg H_2O/L of delivered gas at 30°C

An HME is not appropriate for patients with thick, copious or bloody secretions (since secretions rapidly contaminate and block the HME). Patients with hypothermia are better treated with active humidification and the additional dead space associated with an HME might be disadvantageous in patients who are experiencing difficulty weaning from ventilation. In patients with large air leaks (e.g. those with a large bronchopleurocutaneous fistula) an HME is not ideal, since significant quantities of humidified gas are lost from the chest and not recycled by the HME.

An HME will remove nebulised drugs if administered at a site nearer to the ventilator than the HME. Repeated nebulisation at a site nearer to the patient than the HME can cause waterlogging of the HME with significantly increased resistance.

2.38 A ventilated 72-year-old man has *Pseudomonas aeruginosa* cultured from his sputum. He is apyrexial and has some minor bi-basal consolidation on chest X-ray which appears to have improved over the last few days. His sputum is green and there are some polymorphs in it on microscopy (++). There is some discussion about the need to treat this organism in this man at this time. It is suggested by the ICU registrar that bronchoscopy might clarify the need for treatment.

What does he mean?
The diagnosis of nosocomial bacterial pneumonia in ventilated patients remains a problem. Isolation of bacteria in the sputum may only represent colonisation. The association with pus cells may simply imply bronchitis (infection limited to the bronchus) rather than pneumonia.

Identification of significant numbers of bacteria in the distal airway is currently the clinical diagnostic method of choice (biopsy is impractical but does represent a 'gold standard', and bronchoscopy is required to get to the distal airways.

MINI-TUTORIAL

The development of new infiltrates on chest X-ray, neutrophilia and pyrexia are supportive evidence of pulmonary infection but are non-specific and can occur for reasons other than pneumonia.

Invasive techniques have been developed to assist with the diagnosis of pneumonia in ventilated patients. These methods depend on the observation that large numbers of bacteria present in distal airways are associated with bacteria in lung tissue and histological pneumonia.

The two most widely used methods are broncho-alveolar lavage (BAL) and protected specimen brush (PSB). Both require bronchoscopy and quantitative bacterial culture. It appears that either method has similar sensitivity. Since BAL results in a larger specimen this can also be examined (at the time of bronchoscopy) for the presence of white cells with intracellular bacteria, which are additional indicators of pulmonary infection.

Prior antibiotic treatment interferes with the sensitivity and specificity of any lower airway sampling technique.

Baker AM, Bowton DL, Haponik EF. Decision making in nosocomial pneumonia. An analytic approach to the interpretation of quantitative bronchoscopic cultures. *Chest* 1995; **107**: 85–95.

Chastre J, Fagon J-Y, Bornet-Lecso M, Calvat S, Dombret M-C, Khani R, Basset F, Gibert C. Evaluation of bronchoscopic techniques for the diagnosis of nosocomial pneumonia. *Am. J. Respir. Crit. Care Med.* 1995; **152**: 231–40.

Torres A, el Ebiary M, Padro L, Gonzalez J, de la Bellacasa JP, Ramirez J, Xaubet A, Ferrer M, Rodriguez-Roisin R. Validation of different techniques for the diagnosis of ventilator-associated pneumonia. Comparison with immediate postmortem pulmonary biopsy. *Am. J. Respir. Crit. Care Med.* 1994; **149**(2 Pt 1): 324–31.

3

Haemodynamics

NOTE:

		Normal range	
CI	cardiac index	(2.5–4.0	l/min/m^2)
SVRI	systemic vascular resistance index	(1970–2390	DS m^2/cm^5)
PVRI	pulmonary vascular resistance index	(225–315	DS m^2/cm^5)
LVSWI	left ventricular stroke work index	(50–62	g/m^2)
CVP	central venous pressure		
PAWP	pulmonary artery wedge pressure		

MINI-TUTORIAL

Causes of hypotension can be determined by considering three components:

- Poor head of pressure to fill pump (low CVP/PCWP).
- Poor pump function (e.g. poor muscle, failure of valves, tamponade or ineffective rate).
- Low downstream resistance (low systemic vascular resistance) (e.g. sepsis, epidural local anaesthetic).

These basic concepts can be applied to the cardiovascular system and represent a very simple but clear way to think about hypotension.

Defining 'normal' values for CVP and PCWP is difficult. Judging in individual patients with reference to blood pressure, cardiac output, stroke volume and urine output is best.

In general terms sick patients require values of CVP/PCWP above 12 mmHg (particularly in the presence of oliguria) and if above 18 mmHg then they may be at risk of pulmonary oedema.

3.1 A 67-year-old man is admitted to ICU in pulmonary oedema and hypotension. His ECG is unchanged from a previous trace and his CK-MB is within normal range. A pulmonary artery catheter is inserted and data collected. His haemodynamic results (below) are shown to you:

SBP	75	mmHg
MBP	60	mmHg
CI	2.15	l/min/m^2
SVRI	3407	DS m^2/cm^5
PVRI	171	DS m^2/cm^5
LVSWI	25.0	g/m^2
CVP	8	mmHg
PAWP	17	mmHg

(a) What abnormalities are present?

Hypotension, low cardiac output, high systemic vascular resistance and low left ventricular stroke work index (LVSWI) – a measure of contractility – is characteristic of cardiogenic shock due to left ventricular failure.

(b) What treatment do you suggest?

Left ventricular filling appears adequate (PCWP 17). Cardiac output may be enhanced by dobutamine, but where there is critical coronary artery stenosis cardiac output may fall further in response to dobutamine, since the increased myocardial oxygen demand induced by the inotropic effect of dobutamine cannot be satisfied and regional myocardial dysfunction is exacerbated. Intra-aortic balloon pumping should improve both cardiac output and myocardial perfusion, and may be indicated.

3.2 A 74-year-old man with severe pancreatitis is admitted to the ICU. He has been given fluid on the ward and has required intermittent intravenous metaraminol while lines were inserted. Now he has some haemodynamic results:

SBP	75	mmHg
MBP	42	mmHg
CI	1.55	l/min/m^2
SVRI	3507	DS m^2/cm^5
PVRI	277	DS m^2/cm^5
LVSWI	11.0	g/m^2
CVP	2	mmHg
PAWP	7	mmHg

What do you consider to be the cause of his hypotension?
The hypotension in this case is clearly related to hypovolaemia. The cardiac index is low, systemic vascular resistance high and both the CVP and PCWP are low.

MINI-TUTORIAL

Following rapid intravascular fluid infusion (challenge) the response of the CVP (and PCWP) is observed. Failure to rise following fluid challenge suggests continuing hypovolaemia, while a maintained rise in response to fluid challenge suggests that adequate fluid volume has been achieved (a marked rise suggests that the patient has left ventricular diastolic failure and is liable to develop pulmonary oedema if fluid is given in large volume or rapidly).

In addition, increase of stroke volume in response to fluid challenge supports the contention that the patient is hypovolaemic, while failure of the stroke volume to rise in response to fluid challenge suggests adequate fluid loading.

Note: beware dogmatic interpretation of haemodynamic data obtained from a patient who has received vasoconstrictors (such as metaraminol) shortly before measurements are taken; the measured SVRI will probably reflect the drug effect rather than the underlying clinical condition.

3.3 A patient with empyema returns to ICU following thoracoplasty. A pulmonary artery catheter has been inserted. The patient is hypotensive and the first haemodynamic results (below) are shown to you:

SBP	85	mmHg
MBP	62	mmHg
CI	3.15	l/min/m^2
SVRI	707	DS m^2/cm^5
PVRI	371	DS m^2/cm^5
LVSWI	31.0	g/m^2
CVP	6	mmHg
PAWP	9	mmHg

(a) What major problems are suggested by these data?
A picture of high cardiac output, low systemic vascular resistance and somewhat low left ventricular stroke work index (LVSWI) – a measure

of contractility – is characteristic of septic shock. Although contractility is reduced (sometimes markedly), cardiac output is increased or maintained because afterload is reduced.

(b) What treatment do you suggest?
A CVP or PCWP of at least 12–15 cm H_2O is required for optimal cardiac performance in sick hypotensive, oliguric patients. Fluid should be administered initially to increase the PCWP to 15 cm H_2O, which (with appropriate antibiotics) may be all the treatment that is required to achieve adequate blood pressure, perfusion and urine output.

3.4 A 34-year-old woman has septic shock due to faecal peritonitis. On the previous shift she became hypotensive and oliguric and was found to have a low CVP and PCWP. Consequently she was given an infusion of colloid.
 She remains hypotensive and you are asked what you want to do about it. Recent haemodynamic results are to hand:

SBP	69	mmHg
MBP	55	mmHg
CI	3.45	l/min/m²
SVRI	637	DS m²/cm⁵
PVRI	265	DS m²/cm⁵
LVSWI	23.0	g/m²
CVP	12	mmHg
PAWP	15	mmHg

(a) What major problems are suggested by this data?
Hypotension, low systemic vascular resistance, high cardiac index and adequate left ventricular filling pressure (PAWP). The vascular resistance requires to be increased to achieve an adequate blood pressure to maintain organ perfusion and particularly urine output.

(b) What treatment do you suggest?
A vasoconstrictor and/or inotrope infusion is indicated. The choice will depend upon local preference (see below).

MINI-TUTORIAL

Noradrenaline has less β_1 action at a given dose than does adrenaline. Noradrenaline predominantly has an α action, which results in vasoconstriction. Excessive doses increase afterload and reduce cardiac index, which is not desired; consequently, haemodynamic monitoring is advisable.

Adrenaline generally exhibits both α and β actions and would be expected to increase systemic vascular resistance in a patient with septic shock. A rise in plasma lactate is an expected effect when adrenaline infusion is used in patients with sepsis (see below).

Dopamine in higher dose (> 5 μg/kg/min) generally exhibits both β and α adrenergic effect to variable degree.

Dobutamine increases cardiac index but may further decrease vascular resistance and consequently not result in a blood pressure rise.

All of these agents are used in different ICUs to treat patients with sepsis. There is currently no consensus which is the best choice of inotrope in septic patients with hypotension unresponsive to fluids.

In patients with sepsis requiring inotrope support the effect of adrenaline has been compared to that of dopamine. Cardiac index and oxygen delivery increased in both treatment groups. Lactate levels fell in those treated with dopamine but rose significantly in those treated with adrenaline.

Lactate rises are not associated with treatment with noradrenaline, dobutamine or dopamine.

Adrenaline administered to volunteers results in a small rise in plasma lactate, probably mediated by a β_2 effect. This appears to be similar to the effect seen with salbutamol infusion.

Day NP, Phu NH, Bethell DP, Mai NT, Chau TT, Hien TT, White NJ. The effects of dopamine and adrenaline infusions on acid-base balance and systemic haemodynamics in severe infection. *Lancet* 1996; **348**(9022): 219–23.

3.5 A 77-year-old woman is being managed in intensive care following major surgery for a pharyngeal tumour. She weighs 76 kg and since surgery has passed an average of 80 ml of urine per hour and in the last hour has passed 70 ml.

SBP	125	mmHg
MBP	90	mmHg
CVP	7	mmHg

Her low CVP is pointed out to you and you are asked if you want to give her some intravenous fluid.

What will you do?
Explain that the urine output and blood pressure in this patient are adequate and that giving fluid simply with the aim of achieving a particular level of CVP (or PAWP) is not indicated.

3.6 A 68-year-old man has been admitted to coronary care following what appears to be a reasonably large inferior myocardial infarction. He has been hypotensive for the last 12 hours (since shortly after admission) and has passed only 30 ml of urine despite having been started on dopamine (3 μg/kg/min) and frusemide 80 mg iv. It is now 2 a.m. and you are asked by the night resident to advise what to do about his urine output.

SBP	69	mmHg
MBP	52	mmHg
CVP	28	mmHg

(a) What are the possible causes of this situation?
Patients with inferior myocardial infarction do not usually infarct so much left ventricle that they develop cardiogenic shock (unless they have had previous myocardial damage). The right ventricle may be severely compromised by right ventricular infarction, and right ventricular failure may occur (indicated by a high CVP) with severe under filling of the left ventricle (indicated by a low PCWP). The alternative is that he has left ventricular failure causing cardiogenic shock.

(b) What investigations do you suggest?
A pulmonary artery catheter or echocardiogram will help to elucidate the situation.

A pulmonary artery catheter is inserted and the following results are obtained.

CI	1.85	l/min/m^2
SVRI	3227	DS m^2/cm^5
PVRI	271	DS m^2/cm^5
LVSWI	17.0	g/m^2
CVP	24	mmHg
PAWP	6	mmHg

(c) What do these results tell you?

In a patient with cardiogenic shock a high CVP with a low PCWP is characteristic of cardiogenic shock due to right ventricular failure (this would occur in right ventricular myocardial infarction, as in this case, or massive pulmonary embolism). Fluid loading is indicated and is often remarkably effective.

3.7 A 67-year-old man with known tight left main coronary artery stenosis presents with pulmonary oedema and hypotension (60/45). He has poor peripheral perfusion, and his peripheries are cold and clammy. He has had a catheter inserted but is anuric. The ECG shows ischaemic changes but no signs of acute infarction, and his CK-MB is not raised. In view of his hypotension a dobutamine infusion has been initiated in the Emergency department and is now on 20 μg/kg/min. His clinical state is unchanged.

The Emergency registrar suggests that this is cardiogenic shock and that the outlook is hopeless.

What do you think?

It appears that this man has not infarcted his myocardium (there are no ECG changes and no CK-MB rise to suggest this) and therefore if flow is restored to the ischaemic myocardium the pulmonary oedema, hypotension and poor perfusion should resolve.

There are two approaches to improve coronary blood flow through a tight stenosis. One is to increase the perfusion pressure (diastolic blood pressure) by the use of vasoconstrictors (e.g. metaraminol or noradrenaline), the other is to insert an intra-aortic balloon pump (IABP). Either is appropriate.

MINI-TUTORIAL

Dobutamine is commonly employed in patients with cardiogenic shock. However, the vasodilation (which may further drop diastolic coronary perfusion pressure) associated with dobutamine, together with increased oxygen demand in ischaemic tissue distal to a severe fixed obstruction caused by the dobutamine, may actually exacerbate the situation and cause clinical deterioration. This is the basis of the dobutamine stress echocardiography test, which identifies the presence of significant coronary arterial stenosis. Dobutamine infusion is used in this test to induce ischaemia in the myocardium distal to the stenosis. This is identified by reduced contractility, which is seen as wall motion abnormality on echocardiography. Ceasing the dobutamine infusion is an important diagnostic move in these patients and may result in resolution of the clinical situation (before other measures are instituted). High doses of GTN can also cause significant hypotension and similarly discontinuation may also be associated with beneficial clinical effects. Intravascular hypovolaemia following a massive diuresis in response to an excessively generous dose of frusemide given in the Emergency department may be a further factor which requires consideration in patients who become hypotensive after presenting with pulmonary oedema.

3.8 A patient with significant coronary artery disease has been admitted to ICU for post-operative monitoring following a colectomy. He becomes hypotensive following an epidural bolus. Despite being given fluid rapidly he remains hypotensive after 5 minutes and is observed to have some ST segment depression on a V5 ECG trace. The ICU specialist asks you to 'give some aramine'.

How will you make it up, and how much will you give?
Metaraminol (Aramine) comes as 10 mg in 1 ml. It needs diluting usually to 10 ml (1 mg/ml) and is then given ½ to 1 ml intravenously. Do NOT give 10 mg as severe hypertension is likely to occur.

4

Urine output

Since so many questions posed to juniors in the Intensive Care Unit relate to oliguria this is presented as a separate chapter, although the concepts overlap with haemodynamics.

4.1 You are asked to see a 78-year-old man on the medical ward with pneumonia who is oliguric. He has a blood pressure of 110/70 and a pulse rate of 112. His skin turgor is reduced and his tongue appears dry. He says he is thirsty. He has a central line *in situ* and the most recent CVP is recorded as 6 cm H_2O. The intern says that he doesn't think he is 'dry', since his CVP is normal.

Do you agree?
No. In normal individuals the CVP is said to be 3–5 cm H_2O but in clinical practice it is clear that most patients require higher CVP values to maintain good urine output (this is particularly true in older patients with ventricular hypertrophy and reduced cardiac compliance). In patients who are oliguric in the intensive care unit it is generally necessary to increase the CVP (or PCWP) to at least 15 cm H_2O before accepting that the patient is not hypovolaemic.

MINI-TUTORIAL

It is necessary to be aware of the relationship between pressure readings when fluid manometry is used (cm H_2O) and when pressure transducers are used (mmHg). *7.4 mmHg is equivalent to 10 cm of water pressure* (since mercury density is 13.6 g/cm^3).
  This is particularly relevant when fluid manometry is used outside the ICU and pressure transducers are used in the ICU, with patients moving between each area.

4.2 You are asked to review a 69-year-old man who has had an elective infra-renal aortic aneurysm repair and has become anuric. An extract from his progress chart is shown below:

	Pulse rate	Systolic BP	CVP	Urine output
1000	90	140	12	60
1100	95	130	14	50
1200	90	135	15	80
0100	90	120	13	0
0200	90	140	15	0
0300	94	145	16	0
0400	90	130	16	0

(a) What is the most likely cause for this oliguria?
Absolute and sudden cessation of good urine flow, in the absence of hypotension, is almost always due to catheter blockage.

(b) Are there any investigations you would wish to perform?
The abdomen should be palpated and the catheter washed out to diagnose and rectify the problem.

   Although renal failure due to acute onset chronic renal disease may occur, especially if there is operative hypotension or supra-renal aortic clamping, this is only considered after pre-renal failure – a much more common and more simply treated problem – is excluded.

4.3 A 74-year-old patient with known chronic renal failure presents with pancreatitis. During his first hours in the ICU (during which he received N/saline at 80 ml/h) his urine output remained poor. You have just come on duty and are immediately asked what you want to do about his urine output. An extract from his progress chart is shown below:

	Pulse rate	Mean BP	CVP	Urine output
1000	90	70	2	14
1100	95	80	4	8
1200	90	60	5	5
0100	90	65	5	0
0200	90	60	5	4
0300	94	70	5	0
0400	90	65	5	0

(a) What is the most likely cause for this oliguria?

This patient has a low CVP throughout. Pancreatitis is associated with a marked loss of fluid from the intravascular space. Most patients will need colloid and/or blood to keep up their urine output. Low filling pressure MUST be rectified rapidly in the face of oliguria. To permit such a situation to persist for 6 hours, as in this case, suggests inadequate management and may condemn the patient to acute renal failure.

(b) Are there any investigations you would wish to perform?
Physical examination and checking the catheter is always appropriate. The response of the CVP, blood pressure and urine output to a 500 ml bolus of colloid given rapidly intravenously is the most important information in this situation.

4.4 The night intern asks you to see a 53-year-old alcoholic man on the medical ward. He has been admitted with a chest infection and has become increasingly pyrexial and confused overnight. Four hours ago he was given 40 mg of frusemide iv which resulted in 46 ml of urine (see chart below), but oliguria has persisted:

CVP	Systolic BP	Mean BP	Pulse rate	Urine output
8	110	78	72	20
7	112	82	73	46
4	112	83	75	12
4	110	80	77	10
3	115	80	76	8

The intern is worried that 40 mg of frusemide has not had a lasting effect and asks if a bigger dose or an infusion would be best. What will you advise him?
Diuretic (including dopamine) given in the face of low circulating volume may transiently increase urine output but the oliguria is an appropriate physiological response to the reduced circulating volume. In this situation diuretic treatment is inappropriate and is probably detrimental.

Sick patients who are oliguric will usually require their CVP to be at least 12–15 mmHg (certainly you should not presume that they are 'well filled' below this value of CVP if they are oliguric).

This patient requires fluid to raise CVP, and an increase in urine output would then be expected.

4.5 You are called to review a 67-year-old man who is ventilated for an exacerbation of COAD because of poor urine output:

CVP	Systolic BP	Mean BP	Pulse rate	Urine output
18	120	75	81	20
17	122	80	86	16
17	112	83	90	15
20	110	80	82	12
18	115	83	89	12

(a) What is your evaluation of his oliguria?
There is no evidence on this data that there is inadequate circulating volume (the CVP is high throughout). The blood pressure appears adequate to support urine output (a mean pressure of 80 should be adequate). The urine flow seems to be sluggish for no obvious cause.

(b) What treatment will you suggest for the oliguria?
A diuretic is appropriate in this situation, particularly in the face of clinical signs of fluid overload.

4.6 A 72-year-old man is admitted to ICU following a Hartmann's procedure for faecal peritonitis. He is known to have coronary artery disease and was observed to develop ST segment depression during his anaesthetic.
  He remains intubated and six hours after admission your attention is drawn to his poor urine output:

CVP	Systolic BP	Mean BP	Pulse rate	Urine output
16	80	65	105	20
17	75	60	110	16
20	75	60	117	12
24	75	62	115	8
23	76	60	112	10

(a) What is your assessment of the data presented?
There is no evidence on this data that there is inadequate circulating volume (the CVP is high throughout).
  The blood pressure appears inadequate to support urine output. Patients require an adequate blood pressure to maintain urine output. The satisfactory value varies between patients. A value of 60 can be

adequate in a vasodilated patient but is rarely associated with good urine output in a vasoconstricted (cold, clammy, shut down) patient.

Patients who have a history of hypertension may require a higher blood pressure than previously normotensive patients. Aiming for a mean blood pressure of 80 is probably appropriate in oliguric patients.

(b) Is intravenous frusemide appropriate?
No. A diuretic is inappropriate in this situation. It is unlikely to have an effect in the face of hypotension and it indicates that the reason for the oliguria has not been appreciated. Either an inotrope or vasoactive agent is indicated depending on the clinical evaluation and further investigations (such as a pulmonary artery catheter or echocardiogram).

4.7 A 78-year-old woman remains in ICU following coronary artery bypass. Her operation was two days ago and she is now extubated, but has required 60% oxygen and has significant left lower lobe consolidation. You observe that she is oliguric and review her chart:

CVP	Systolic BP	Mean BP	Pulse rate	Urine output
15	110	70	72	40
17	80	65	167	16
19	69	55	175	4
19	65	55	177	5
21	67	52	189	2

(a) What is your assessment of the data presented?
There is no evidence on this data that there is inadequate circulating volume (the CVP is high throughout).

The blood pressure appears inadequate to support urine output.

This may be due to either poor cardiac output or low vascular resistance. Poor cardiac output can be due to either ventricular failure or an ineffective rate. Here there is evidence of an inappropriately rapid rate. A variable rate between 160 and 200 is likely to be atrial fibrillation (AF). In this case an ECG revealed that the rapid rate was caused by uncontrolled AF.

(b) How do you suggest the oliguria be treated?
The rapid AF appears to be causing significant haemodynamic compromise. Where there is significant haemodynamic compromise DC cardioversion is appropriate – otherwise drug treatment, either with the aim of reverting to sinus rhythm (e.g. amiodarone) or controlling the rate (e.g. digoxin) is indicated.

4.8 A 75-year-old woman passes minimal urine following a difficult abdomino-perineal resection of the rectum. She is known to have only one functioning kidney (the other having been removed).
   Her blood pressure and volume status appear satisfactory.

What investigation will you arrange?
Ruling out obstruction as the cause of renal failure is always important. This is most easily done by a renal ultrasound scan. In this patient obstruction is likely, since she has undergone pelvic surgery where difficulties were encountered.

4.9 A 70-year-old man returns to ICU after a difficult abdominal aortic aneurysm repair following a posterior rupture. He initially puts out good urine in ICU (60, 85, 70, 55 ml over the first 4 hours) but then becomes oliguric (10 ml/h then 2 ml/h of urine then none). His blood pressure remains at between 120 and 160 mmHg systolic. His CVP is 17 mmHg and PCWP is 18 mmHg. The surgical registrar suggests an urgent renal angiogram.

(a) Do you agree?
No.

(b) What is the most likely cause for this oliguria?
This man appears to have a good pre-load and is not obstructed. Early in the post-operative course intra-abdominal bleeding with high intra-abdominal pressures is relatively common. High pressures correlate with oliguria.

(c) Are there any investigations you would wish to perform?
Intra-abdominal pressure is measured by connecting a manometer to the urinary catheter. Fifty millilitres of saline is injected into the bladder and the pressure is then measured using the symphysis pubis as the zero point.

(d) What treatment will you suggest?

When high pressures are demonstrated, patients need to be returned to theatre and the abdomen decompressed – when the pressure is reduced the urine starts to flow almost immediately. Failure to decompress the abdomen results in needless renal failure.

Platell CF, Hall J, Clarke G, Lawrence-Brown M. Intra-abdominal pressure and renal function after surgery to the abdominal aorta. *Aust. N. Z. J. Surg.* 1990; **60**(3): 213–16.

4.10 You are admitting a 67-year-old man who has become acutely oliguric and hyperkalaemic (K+ 7.2 mmol/l). He has a history of hypertension, cardiac failure, peripheral vascular disease and gout. He is currently hypotensive 65/40 and has poor skin turgor. He is treated with lisinopril, indomethacin and frusemide.

The medical registrar suggests that his medication might be a factor in his renal failure.

What do you think?

Yes. In patients with poor renal perfusion (and consequently low glomerular filtration pressure) both non-steroidal anti-inflammatory drugs (NSAIDs) and ACE inhibitors can provoke renal failure. Diuretics can result in intravascular volume depletion, and this compounds poor renal perfusion and the renal effects of the other drugs.

MINI-TUTORIAL

Under normal conditions, NSAIDs have relatively little effect on the kidney because of low renal production of prostaglandins. However, in the presence of renal hypoperfusion in which local synthesis of vasodilator prostaglandins is increased to protect the glomerular haemodynamics and to maintain appropriate renal tubular transport of fluid and electrolytes, inhibition of prostaglandin synthesis by NSAIDs can lead to vasoconstrictive acute renal failure.

In the face of decreased glomerular filtration pressure glomerular filtration becomes critically dependent on angiotensin II-mediated efferent vascular tone. Renal artery stenosis or severe depletion of circulating volume (e.g. acute diarrhoea or diuretic therapy) predispose patients treated with angiotensin converting enzyme (ACE) inhibitors to develop acute renal failure (ARF).

Following withdrawal of either or both drugs, recovery of renal function can be anticipated even when a period of dialysis or haemofiltration is required.

Pugliese F, Cinotti GA. Nonsteroidal anti-inflammatory drugs (NSAIDs) and the
   kidney. *Nephrol Dial. Transplant.* 1997; **12**(3): 386–8.
Wynckel A, Ebikili B, Melin JP, Randoux C, Lavaud S, Chanard J. Long-term
   follow-up of acute renal failure caused by angiotensin converting enzyme
   inhibitors. *Am. J. Hypertens.* 1998; **11**(9): 1080–6.

**4.11 You are caring for a patient who has developed oliguric
renal failure. It has been decided that haemofiltration should be
initiated. Before anything is organised the medical registrar
arrives and asks why you are haemofiltrating the patient rather
than haemodialysing him.**

What reasons will you give?

Haemofiltration is performed continuously, rather than haemodialysis, which is performed intermittently. Haemodialysis is designed
to clear all the metabolites and achieve all the required fluid shifts
within a short time (3–4 hours). Such rapid shifts are poorly tolerated
by sick ICU patients (hypertonic dialysate and the use of acetate as a
dialysate buffer are additional factors which may contribute to poor
tolerance); hence the widespread use of continuous systems in intensive care units.

MINI-TUTORIAL

In haemofiltration blood is passed, at pressure, over a permeable
membrane through which fluid and solutes pass as a result of hydro-
static forces (Fig. 4.1). Since fluid loss through the filter is large (about
1 litre/h) fluid and solute replacement is required. Urea, creatinine, etc.
are not replaced and are consequently cleared.

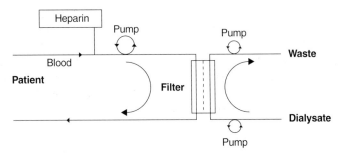

Fig. 4.1

The flow for haemofiltration is either arterial to venous (AV), with the arterial pressure driving the blood flow, or is venous to venous (VV), the blood flow being driven by a pump. Generally VV is preferred, since it is more reliable and avoids the complications associated with prolonged cannulation of large arteries.

While clearance of creatinine and urea is reasonable on CVVH (continuous veno-venous haemofiltration), a number of adaptations have been made to improve clearance. These include:

- Administration of replacement fluids to the blood before the filter (predilution). This reduces the plasma concentration of urea, which encourages movement of urea from red cells and reduces the oncotic pressure, which results in increased ultrafiltration.
- Adding a countercurrent dialysate flow to the filtrate side of the filter increases solute removal by diffusion (addition of dialysate is denoted by a 'D' – hence CVVHD).

The large fluid fluxes of haemofiltration necessitate close observation of fluid balance and frequent bag changes. It has been found that restricting the ultrafiltrate flow by pumping it rather than permitting it to flow freely permits more control.

Large bore double lumen central venous catheters are used for CVVH with the blood being pumped through the filter (flow rates of 100–150 ml/min are generally recommended). Where diafiltration is employed, dialysate flows of 1–2 litres per hour are usual.

By controlling both dialysate input and filter output a desired overall (including IV input) fluid balance can be achieved (e.g. 100 ml negative per hour).

4.12 An APTT (activated partial thromboplastin time) has been performed at 9 p.m. for a patient on continuous veno-venous haemodiafiltration. The result is 146 seconds.

Do you wish to alter the rate of heparin infusion?

It depends. It is important to be clear from where this blood sample has been obtained. If it has been taken from the haemofiltration circuit beyond the point that the heparin is being infused then the result is acceptable (the aim is to achieve good anti-coagulation in the circuit). If the sample was taken from the circuit before the heparin infusion or from a venous stab then the patient is over anti-coagulated and a reduction in the rate of heparin infusion is indicated.

MINI-TUTORIAL

Coagulation tests can be taken from arterial lines which are being flushed with heparin, but a reasonable volume of blood should be discarded (> 5 ml) before the sample for analysis is taken. Even so, confusing results still occur, and clotting results which seem odd should be repeated if taken from an arterial line.

NB: Some units use heparin in the saline flush for arterial lines; others do not. The evidence on this matter remains unclear.

4.13 Your attention is drawn to a lactate result of 5.6 mmol/l. The patient, who is in ICU with systemic vasculitis, has been reasonably haemodynamically stable with a mean blood pressure of around 75 mmHg (without inotropes). He has not been systemically hypoxic and does not have clinical signs of sepsis. He is on continuous haemodiafiltration for oliguric renal failure. The physician is concerned that the lactate indicates that the patient has tissue hypoxia and thinks that 'something needs to be done'.

What do you think?

Standard haemofiltration replacement (and dialysis) fluid contains lactate rather than bicarbonate as the anion. There is thus a constant infusion of lactate into patients on haemofiltration. Serum lactate levels rise in most sick patients on haemofiltration, particularly when there is hepatic dysfunction. In this situation the increased lactate does not reflect tissue lactate production and is not ominous. Where lactate levels become very high (e.g. above 10 mmol/l) it is reasonable to consider using a bicarbonate-containing haemofiltration fluid.

5

Sepsis

5.1 A 40-year-old woman is admitted to intensive care after drainage of a hepatic abscess in another hospital. The surgical note reports that a corrugated drain was placed into the abscess cavity. She was given metronidazole and gentamicin intravenously in theatre, and this has been continued subsequently. Culture has grown a pure growth of *Bacteroides fragillis*.

In the four days following surgery the patient has not progressed well. The white cell count has risen to $23 \times 10^9/l$ (having been $13 \times 10^9/l$ pre-operatively). She is still ventilated and oxygenation has deteriorated (she is now on 80% oxygen). Her X-ray shows significant bi-basal consolidation. Although her creatinine was normal pre-operatively she is now oliguric and has a creatinine of 420 μmol/l. The referring surgeon thinks that pneumonia is the cause of her deterioration.

While awaiting the surgeon you are asked what you think the problem might be and what initial investigation is required.

What will you say?

This lady has had an operation which should have made her much better, although it is possible that she could have become transiently worse due to bacteraemia during drainage. This is not the case and you must be suspicious. In all cases where patients fail to improve, particularly where there are signs of sepsis and where there is progressive organ failure, an infected collection requires exclusion.

A CT scan of the abdomen is the most appropriate investigation in this case (Fig. 5.1). It rapidly confirms that the abscess is still present and that the drain is sitting laterally to the abscess.

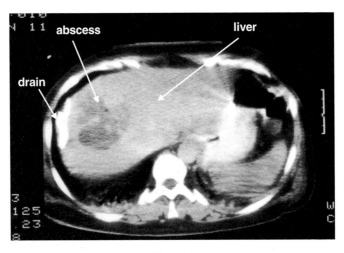

Fig. 5.1

MINI-TUTORIAL

In almost all cases where there is intra-abdominal pathology with collection of infected material there will be consolidation at the lung bases. It is easy to ascribe deterioration of the patient to this (and surgeons will usually try); however, nosocomial pneumonia is very rarely the cause of progressive multi-organ failure, while intra-abdominal collection is a well recognised cause.

Continual investigation to track down the source of sepsis is extremely important in intensive care patients who are not improving and are developing progressive organ failure. In most cases the abdominal cavity is the source.

5.2 A 56-year-old diabetic man is admitted to the ICU due to sepsis. He was noted to have cloudy urine on admission to ICU and microscopy revealed numerous Gram-negative bacilli in his urine. A diagnosis of urinary tract infection was made and he was treated with gentamicin to which *E. coli*, which was subsequently isolated, is sensitive.

Despite the antibiotic treatment he continues to deteriorate. He remains intubated and requires a significant dose of noradrenaline (0.5 μ/kg/min) to maintain his blood pressure. His blood sugar levels are difficult to control with large doses of intravenous insulin.

The diabetic physician asks you if you are sure that his clinical state is explained by his urinary tract infection.

What will you say?
No, you should not be sure at all.

Systemic sepsis associated with simple urinary tract infection can cause significant haemodynamic effect, but classically responds rapidly to treatment. Neither have any investigations been done to exclude urinary obstruction (infection in obstructed urine has much more profound effects than in free-flowing urine).

Failure to respond should rapidly raise the possibility of obstructed infected urine or to another cause for the clinical picture (e.g. pancreatitis).

An ultrasound or CT scan would help to exclude obstruction and collection. In this case a CT was performed and showed absence of the left kidney which is replaced by gas and pus (Fig. 5.2). Severe renal infection complicated by papillary necrosis is a particular risk in diabetic patients.

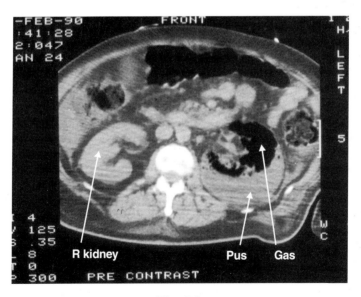

Fig. 5.2

6
Antibiotics

It is important to consider hospital antibiotic resistance patterns in your antibiotic choices and also to establish whether there is a written hospital antibiotic prescribing policy for various clinical indications. The widespread development of multi-resistant organisms is felt to be associated with liberal antibiotic usage, and consequently there is pressure to moderate antibiotic prescribing.

6.1 A 73-year-old lady required a laparotomy for diverticular disease at which a perforation with significant faecal soiling of the peritoneum was found and lavaged. She now returns to ICU following a Hartmann's procedure and is found to be hypotensive and pyrexial. She appears to have received no antibiotics in theatre. The surgeon mentions he would like her to have some antibiotics.

Suggest an appropriate antibiotic regimen.
Abscess formation in faeculent peritonitis results from Gram-negative bacilli, anaerobic bacilli and enterococcus (previously termed *Streptococcus faecalis*). All of these must be covered. Either cefotaxime or gentamicin are appropriate for Gram-negative bacilli. Metronidazole is required for anaerobes. Amoxycillin is required for *Enterococcus faecalis* cover – all cephalosporins cover Enterococcus poorly. Imipenem will cover all three types of organism (Gram-negative bacilli, anaerobic bacilli and enterococcus) but is costly and is not currently recommended first line treatment. Ticarcillin/clavulinic acid (Timentin) is an alternative choice.

6.2 A 66-year-old patient with COAD who has been in hospital for four weeks following a laparotomy now has a right lower lobe pneumonia and is becoming increasingly sick. Blood cultures have been taken and it is suggested that she be given antibiotics.

What will you prescribe?
This is likely to be a nosocomial pneumonia. Following abdominal surgery Gram-negative organisms will be the most probable pathogens, but anaerobic cover is also indicated. Third generation cephalosporin with metronidazole would be appropriate. Sputum culture should be obtained (if possible) before antibiotics are initiated and the results of both blood and sputum culture should be obtained as soon as they are available. Antibiotic treatment may require to be adjusted in the light of culture results.

MINI-TUTORIAL

In any patient who has been in hospital for some time the possibility that they have become colonised and subsequently infected by resistant organisms (most commonly methicillin-resistant *Staphylococcus aureus*: MRSA) should be seriously considered. Enquiry about other infected patients on the ward from which the patient has come may help to determine the risk (if none have it is very unlikely your patient is infected, if several are infected it is highly likely). Identification of Gram-positive cocci on sputum staining will also be highly supportive.

6.3 A previously well 18-year-old student is admitted to ICU with a one-day history of malaise, headache and myalgia. Over the last 6 hours he has become increasingly drowsy and is now unresponsive to pain. On examination he is found to have some dark petechial blotches on his lower legs.

In the Emergency department it is suggested that he should be given some antibiotic before he has a CT scan of his brain and then a lumbar puncture.

Is this a reasonable approach? What antibiotic regimen will you prescribe?
Yes. The clinical picture is consistent with a clinical diagnosis of meningococcal septicaemia. The situation is life-threatening and it is essential that an appropriate antibiotic is administered as soon as possible. Administration should not be delayed while diagnostic tests are performed.

Benzylpenicillin 30 mg/kg intravenously 4 hourly is standard treatment (cefotaxime 2 g 8 hourly is an acceptable alternative).

6.4 An orthopaedic consultant notices that one of his patients in intensive care is on 320 mg of gentamicin once daily. He comments that he used to give 80 mg three times daily and asks you why you are giving such a big dose once.

What will you tell him?
A single daily dose of gentamicin of 5–7 mg/kg is now recommended in adults with normal renal function.

MINI-TUTORIAL

There are a number of rationales for one daily dosing:

- Higher concentrations of aminoglycosides result in more effective bacterial killing.
- Selection of resistant organisms during treatment is less likely when higher concentrations of drug are used.
- Following a bactericidal dose aminoglycosides have been shown to suppress bacterial growth for prolonged periods.
- The overall 'area under the curve' following aminoglycoside dosing is best related to efficacy, rather than the time that the minimum inhibitory concentration is exceeded.
- Nephrotoxicity is reduced when higher doses are given less frequently.

Using the once-daily regimen it is unnecessary to measure peak drug levels (which are assured by the large dose). A single measurement of the plasma concentration 12 hours after the end of the infusion can be used to review the drug dose.
    Lower doses and/or frequency are required in patients with impairment of renal function.

Prins JM, Buller HR *et al*. Once versus thrice daily gentamicin in patients with serious infections. *Lancet* 1993; **341**: 335–3.

6.5 A patient being treated for faecal peritonitis has developed severe diarrhoea. You are asked if you 'want to send a sample to the lab'.

Is this worthwhile and if so what will you request?
Yes, it is worthwhile. A *Clostridium difficile* toxin is probably the most important and useful test to request.

MINI-TUTORIAL

Faecal microscopy is useful to identify parasites (e.g. Giardia, Cryptosporidium, Blastocystis).

Red and white cells can also be identified, which indicates mucosal inflammation.

Culture may identify pathogenic organisms (e.g. Salmonella, Campylobacter, Shigella).

Both faecal microscopy and culture are indicated in community-acquired severe diarrhoea or epidemics, but are not so useful in the isolated case of diarrhoea in the ICU. (Note that even when there is bloody diarrhoea in an ICU patient it is much more likely to be due to bowel ischaemia or other surgical causes rather than to infection).

The vast majority of diarrhoea in the ICU is related to general illness (for which no cause is evident). A serious cause of diarrhoea in ICU patients is pseudomembranous colitis. This is caused by *Clostridium difficile* growth in the bowel and is associated with antibiotic use (classically clindamycin, but in practice most antibiotics). *Clostridium difficile* produces a toxin which causes mucosal damage and diarrhoea. This toxin can be measured in the faeces. Treatment is with metronidazole (oral or intravenous) or oral vancomycin (vancomycin is out of favour since it may encourage the development of vancomycin-resistant enterococcus).

6.6 You receive a sputum culture and sensitivity result for a patient who is intubated following a head injury. He has been intubated for 5 days and is on no antibiotic. The sputum sample was taken as a routine, but subsequently the patient has become febrile. The sputum now appears purulent.

Gram stain

Polymorphs	++
Epithelial cells	–
Gram-positive cocci	–
Gram-positive bacilli	–
Gram-negative cocci	–
Gram-negative bacilli	++

Culture
Enterobacter cloacae

Sensitivities

Amoxycillin	R
Cefotaxime/ceftriaxone	S
Cephalexin	R
Gentamicin	S
Co-trimoxazole	R
Imipenem	S

Which antibiotic will you prescribe?
Either gentamicin or imipenem is appropriate. Gentamicin is significantly cheaper. Although the sensitivity suggests sensitivity to cephalosporin, this is not the best choice since inducible resistance is liable to occur rapidly.

MINI-TUTORIAL

Citrobacter freundi, Enterobacter and Serratia species of bacteria develop 'inducible resistance' to cephalosporins. They are often initially sensitive to third-generation cephalosporins but become resistant after a few days of treatment. This is due to the selection of cephalosporinase-producing bacteria in the bacterial population. If the bacterium is sensitive to gentamicin (as it usually is) this would be a better antibiotic with which to treat since induction of resistance does not occur.

7

Infection control

7.1 You are about to put a central venous line into a patient in the intensive care unit. There are both sulfadiazine-chlorhexidine impregnated catheters and standard (non-impregnated) catheters in the cupboard. The surgical registrar suggests that the impregnated catheter 'doesn't have much effect and costs a lot more'.

Is he correct?
Not really. Impregnated catheters do cost more. There is evidence that they reduce both catheter-associated infection (CAI) and, more importantly, catheter-associated bacteraemia (CAB). There is increasing use of these catheters in high-risk patients (including critically ill patients). The value will depend on underlying catheter infection rates, but since the effects of catheter-associated bacteraemia can be very severe (including endocarditis) the use of impregnated catheters can generally be justified.

MINI-TUTORIAL

Catheter-associated infection (CAI) may be defined as > 15 colony-forming units in the semi-quantitative culture of the catheter tip (the tip is rolled on an agar plate). Catheter-associated bacteraemia (CAB) is defined as isolation of the same organism from the catheter and blood in a patient with sepsis syndrome.

Catheter infection can occur due to migration of bacteria from the catheter–skin interface along the external surface of the catheter (thought to be the major route) or by way of bacterial contamination of the catheter hub and migration down the inside of the catheter.

Evidence in favour of the external route of catheter infection includes:

- A high association with positive external catheter culture and blood infection.
- Skin infection at the insertion site is very highly associated with both catheter and blood infection.
- Barriers, such as silver salt impregnated cuffs, on the external surface of catheters reduce infection rates.

- Topical disinfectants to the insertion site reduce catheter tip infection rates.

Hubs are frequently colonised, particularly in longer term catheterisations.

Coagulase negative staphylococci are the most frequent organisms isolated from infected catheters. Although they are most frequently isolated they do not cause bacteraemia as often as does *Staphylococcus aureus*.

The vast majority of catheter-associated bacteraemias are associated with central lines.

Most studies indicate that jugular venous access is associated with significantly more risk of infection when compared with subclavian venous access.

Anti-microbial coating of catheters can reduce CAI from about 14% to 8%.

Coating of the outer surface of catheters with sulfadiazine-chlorhexidine has been reported to reduce the incidence of CAB (but only the outer surface is coated in the Arrowgard product, so the effectiveness may decline as hub infection becomes more important with time). A meta-analysis of studies by Veenstra *et al.* (1999) supports the contention that these catheters reduce both CAI and CAB in short-term central venous catheterisation.

Catheters impregnated with rifampicin and minocycline also appear to reduce the incidence of CAI and CAB. This effect appears to persist.

When the catheters were directly compared it was found that catheters impregnated with minocycline and rifampicin were less likely than those impregnated with chlorhexidine and silver sulfadiazine to be colonised (7.9% vs. 22.8%, $P < 0.001$), and much less likely to be associated with catheter-related bloodstream infection (0.3% vs. 3.4%, $P < 0.002$).

Darouiche RO, Raad II, Heard SO, Thornby JI, Wenker OC, Gabrielli A, Berg J, Khardori N, Hanna H, Hachem R, Harris RL, Mayhall G. A comparison of two antimicrobial-impregnated central venous catheters. Catheter Study Group. *N. Engl. J. Med.* 1999; **340**(1): 1–8.

Maki DG, Weise CE, Sarafin HW. A semiquantitative culture method for identifying intravenous-catheter-related infection. *N. Engl. J. Med.* 1977; **296**(23): 1305–9.

Veenstra DL, Saint S, Saha S, Lumley T, Sullivan SD. Efficacy of antiseptic-impregnated central venous catheters in preventing catheter-related bloodstream infection: a meta-analysis. *JAMA* 1999; **281**(3): 261–7.

8

Pharmacology

8.1 A 34-year-old woman with multi-system organ dysfunction ('MODS') is recovering in the high-dependency unit after a stormy 6 week course. Her sedation and analgesia were stopped 24 hours ago (morphine and midazolam) after running continuously for three weeks.

She is alert, orientated and breathing spontaneously on oxygen. Over the next 6 hours she becomes extremely anxious, agitated and jittery. She subsequently has a grand mal seizure.

(a) What is the most likely reason that she has had a seizure?
Benzodiazepine withdrawal syndrome is more common, occurs more rapidly and is more severe with short-acting agents such as midazolam rather than longer-acting drugs such as diazepam. Withdrawal is more commonly associated with grand mal seizures and myoclonic jerks than with petit mal seizures.

(b) How should she be managed?
The fit should be controlled with diazepam. Small doses of long-acting benzodiazepine which are progressively decreased will avoid the withdrawal syndrome.

Mets B, Horsell A, Linton DM. Midazolam-induced benzodiazepine withdrawal syndrome. *Anaesthesia* 1991; **46**: 28–9.

8.2 A 59-year-old woman has had a rising creatinine (120 μmol/l up to 235 μmol/l) following thoracotomy. She currently has a wedge pressure of 16 mmHg and a mean arterial blood pressure of 82 mmHg. She has a lax abdomen and has a 1.5 litre positive balance since her surgery. The surgeon is at the bedside and suggests that 'she obviously needs dopamine or will soon be in complete renal failure'.

(a) Is he correct?
No, although dopamine will increase urine output (a diuretic effect) there is no evidence that the incidence of renal failure is reduced by the use of dopamine. A number of studies have been performed,

none of which shows benefit. Although dopamine remains widely used it is important to recognise that there is currently no evidence that dopamine preserves or improves renal function in critically ill patients and continued use is based on tradition rather than on scientific evidence.

Szerlip HM. Renal-dose dopamine: fact and fiction. *Ann. Intern. Med.* 1991; **115**(2): 153-4.

MINI-TUTORIAL

Since dopamine is an important and controversial issue it is useful to be aware of a number of the studies in a little more detail.

Patients undergoing CAGS were treated from induction for 24 hours with either 200 µg/min dopamine or placebo). No improvement in creatinine clearance was evident for the dopamine-treated group.

Myles PS *et al.* Effect of 'Renal dose' dopamine on renal function following cardiac surgery. *Anaes. Intens. Care* 1993; **21**: 56.

In a prospective, randomised, double-blind trial of placebo, dobutamine or dopamine in intensive care patients, more urine output was obtained with dopamine, but improved creatinine clearance was unchanged. Dobutamine resulted in improved creatinine clearance while urine output was not increased over placebo (this study made the important point that increased urine output is not synonymous with improved renal function).

Duke GJ, Briedis JH, Weaver RA. Renal support in critically ill patients: low-dose dopamine or low-dose dobutamine? *Crit. Care Med.* 1994; **22**(12): 1919–25.

After listening to your explanation the surgeon says that in his experience dopamine has worked even if the studies can't show it. He observes that there is no evidence that dopamine does any harm.

(b) Is he correct now?
Unfortunately not. Dopamine has multiple actions, many of which may be undesirable.

MINI-TUTORIAL

Numerous effects have been demonstrated in response to dopamine infusion, many of which are probably unhelpful, especially in the critically ill patient. These include:

- impaired hypoxic pulmonary vasoconstriction
- reduced gastric motility
- endocrine dysfunction (attenuates secretion of growth hormone, reduced circulating T_3)
- immune dysfunction (induction of anergic state)
- decreased gut oxygenation in shock states
- diuresis with inpatients who are hypovolaemic
- reduced respiratory response to hypoxia

Despite years of routine use, dopamine is now falling into disrepute with the failure of trials to demonstrate a benefit together with an increasing recognition of real or potential adverse effects.

Cuthbertson BH, Noble DW. Dopamine in oliguria. *BMJ* 1997; **314**(7082): 690–1.
Van den Berghe G, de Zegher F. Anterior pituitary function during critical illness and dopamine treatment. *Crit. Care Med.* 1996; **24**(9): 1580–90.

8.3 During the ward round there is a discussion about the level of sedation in a particular patient. During the course of this the ICU specialist asks you what problems are caused by over-sedation.

(a) What will you say?
Over-sedation causes cardiorespiratory depression and decreased gastrointestinal mobility. Reduced cough reflex and unnecessary suppression of voluntary respiration as a consequence of excess sedation results in prolongation of mechanical ventilation, with the associated ICU costs and risk of nosocomial infection.

He then goes on to ask you what the problems resulting from under-sedation are.

(b) What will you say now?
Sedation aims to protect patients from the effects of the numerous noxious stimuli to which they are exposed in the ICU and to provide a degree of anxiolysis.

Patients who are inadequately sedated may be hypertensive and tachycardic, and may tolerate mechanical ventilation poorly, resulting in increased respiratory work. As a consequence of distress or disorientation they may remove important therapeutic items, such as an endotracheal tube or central venous lines.

MINI-TUTORIAL

Sedation in ICU is commonly achieved with a combination of benzodiazepine (midazolam is popular) and morphine. There is evidence that the use of propofol is associated with more rapid waking and ventilator weaning; however, propofol is about 2.5 times the cost of midazolam. It may be rational to use propofol in patients who are approaching weaning, rather than for their whole admission. Propofol may also be very useful in patients who become confused and uncooperative during weaning from midazolam.

Barrientos-Vega R *et al.* Prolonged sedation of critically ill patients with midazolam or propofol: impact on weaning and costs. *Crit. Care Med.* 1997; **25**: 33–40.

8.4 On the ward round there is a discussion about the prophylaxis of gastric stress ulceration in patients in intensive care. This has been precipitated by the observation that a patient who is ventilated for a severe infective exacerbation of obstructive airways disease has had some frank blood aspirated from his nasogastric tube. He has had sucralfate 1 g 6 hourly nasogastrically and the ICU registrar states that 'there is evidence that ranitidine is more effective'.

Is he correct?
Yes.

Both sucralfate and ranitidine reduce the incidence of gastric haemorrhage in ICU patients at high risk (i.e. those who are ventilated; unventilated patients have a low risk and it is not recommended they have routine prophylaxis). The overall incidence of haemorrhage has reduced over recent years, probably as a consequence of more rapid and complete resuscitation. A recent multi-centre, randomised, blinded, placebo-controlled trial by the Canadian Critical Care Trials Group concludes that ranitidine is more effective.

MINI-TUTORIAL

In the multi-centre, randomised, blinded, placebo-controlled trial by the Canadian Critical Care Trials Group, sucralfate was compared with ranitidine for the prevention of upper gastrointestinal bleeding in patients who required mechanical ventilation. Significant bleeding occurred in 1.7% of the patients receiving ranitidine vs. 3.8% with sucralfate ($P < 0.05$). A non-significant trend to more pneumonia in patients occurred in

19.1% of those on ranitidine and 16.2% of those on sucralfate (NS). There were no significant differences in the duration of the stay in the ICU, or mortality.

Cook D, Guyatt G, Marshall J, Leasa D, Fuller H, Hall R, Peters S, Rutledge F, Griffith L, McLellan A, Wood G, Kirby A. A comparison of sucralfate and ranitidine for the prevention of upper gastrointestinal bleeding in patients requiring mechanical ventilation. Canadian Critical Care Trials Group. *N. Engl. J. Med.* 1998; **338**(12): 791–7.

8.5 You are caring for a 72-year-old man who has septic shock complicating a necrotising fasciitis. He is requiring high doses of noradrenaline to maintain his blood pressure but his cardiac index is high. The surgeon who has debrided his necrotic leg asks 'Would he benefit from some steroids?'.

What do you think?
The evidence suggests that steroid treatment is unhelpful and is probably detrimental in septic shock.

MINI-TUTORIAL

A number of large studies have failed to show a benefit for high dose steroids in septic shock (e.g. Bone *et al.*, 1987) and a meta-analysis of randomised controlled trials of steroids in septic shock concluded that there is a trend towards detriment in patients with septic shock treated with steroids (Cronin, 1995).

A small number of patients with septic shock (maybe 1%) appear to be unable to increase their cortisol level in response to their stress (Jurney *et al.*, 1987). These patients have a high mortality which appears to be improved by low-dose steroid administration (response to vasopressor has also been seen to improve dramatically in this subset of patients following steroid administration). Measuring cortisol levels (which should be above 500 nmol/l in patients with septic shock) and observing the response to synthetic ACTH ('Synacthen') administration – which should result in a rise of > 200 nmol/l following ACTH administration – may identify patients with inadequate adrenal response who could benefit from temporary low-dose steroid infusion.

Bone RC, Fisher CJ Jr, Clemmer TP, Slotman GJ, Metz CA, Balk RA. A controlled clinical trial of high-dose methylprednisolone in the treatment of severe sepsis and septic shock. *N. Engl. J. Med.* 1987; **317**(11): 653–8.
Cronin L, Cook DJ, Carlet J, Heyland DK, King D, Lansang MA, Fisher CJ Jr. Corticosteroid treatment for sepsis: a critical appraisal and meta-analysis of the literature. *Crit. Care Med.* 1995; **23**(8): 1430–9.

Jurney TH, Cockrell JL Jr, Lindberg JS, Lamiell JM and Wade CE. Spectrum of serum cortisol response to ACTH in ICU patients. Correlation with degree of illness and mortality. *Chest* 1987; **92**: 292–5.

8.6 You have admitted a man with severe ulcerative colitis who requires intubation for respiratory failure secondary to pneumonia. He has been treated with oral prednisolone 60 mg/day and you are asked to give him 'equivalent intravenous steroid '.

What will you prescribe, and how much?
Either hydrocortisone or dexamethasone are appropriate substitutions (prednisolone does not come in an intravenous preparation). There is less tendency to sodium retention with dexamethasone and it is cheaper.

Approximate equivalent doses and duration of action are as follows:

Cortisone	25 mg	8–12 h
Hydrocortisone	20 mg	8–12 h
Prednisolone	5 mg	24 h
Methylprednisolone	4 mg	24 h
Dexamethasone	0.75 mg	36 h

8.7 On a ward round you see a 74-year-old man who has been in ICU for two weeks following a severe pneumonia. The major problem now is that he is very weak and this is preventing him being weaned from ventilation. During discussion about his 'need for muscle' the suggestion is made that growth hormone might help.

Do you think this is a good idea?
Unfortunately not.

Despite encouraging early reports more recent trials have not shown any benefit from treatment with growth hormone in critically ill patients. On the contrary, increased morbidity and mortality appear to result.

MINI-TUTORIAL

There are a number of reasons why growth hormone might be expected to improve muscle bulk and function in critically ill patients. Certainly the effect of growth hormone in athletes is well recognised.

Negative nitrogen balance in critically ill patients is partly attributable to resistance to growth hormone and to reduced production of insulin-like growth factor.

Studies of growth hormone in critically ill patients have suggested that treatment with growth hormone improves nitrogen balance, increases grip strength, increases maximal inspiratory pressures and facilitates weaning from mechanical ventilation. These positive studies have generally been conducted in small numbers of patients and some have not been blinded or randomised.

In a recent large multi-centre study, designed to clarify the situation, growth hormone treatment proved to be associated with increased mortality, increased stay in intensive care and increased time on mechanical ventilation. Hyperglycaemia was more common in patients treated with growth hormone. The current data cannot support the use of growth hormone to promote muscle strength and to facilitate weaning in critically ill patients.

Takala J, Ruokonen E, Webster NR, Nielsen MS, Zandstra DF, Vunderlinckx G, Hinds CJ. Increased mortality associated with growth hormone treatment in critically ill adults. N. Engl. J. Med. 1999; **341**: 785–92.

8.8 You see a 59-year-old man with an acute chest pain consistent with myocardial infarction. He has 1 mm ST segment elevation in leads V2, V3 and V4, but no other abnormality. There is discussion of whether this is adequate ECG evidence to support thrombolytic use.

(a) What do you think?

Generally accepted electrocardiographic criteria for thrombolytic therapy are a presentation within 12 hours of the onset of symptoms of myocardial infarction and ST elevation of 1–2 mm in two or more consecutive leads on the electrocardiogram.

During the same discussion the Emergency registrar states that there is 'clear evidence that TPA is better', but 'we aren't allowed to use it because of the expense'.

(b) Is there a sound basis for this statement?

Not really. There is some experimental evidence that coronary arterial blood flow is re-established faster with TPA (tissue plasminogen activator), but the survival benefits associated with this are not so clear, particularly in patients with smaller infarcts.

MINI-TUTORIAL

The three large comparison trials of different thrombolytic agents and regimens (each including 20 000–40 000 patients) have shown only subtle differences in results:

	Mortality	
	At 5 weeks	
GISSI-2	TPA	SK
	8.9%	8.5%
ISIS-3	TPA	SK
	10.3%	10.6%
	At 30 days	
GUSTO	TPA	SK
	6.3%	7.3%

GUSTO did show narrowly better survival (14% mortality decrease) with TPA, which is thought to be a consequence of more rapid arterial reperfusion associated with use of this agent. The benefit of this effect seems to be greatest where mortality is highest, that is in large or anterior wall infarctions. However, the slightly decreased cardiac mortality associated with TPA use is tempered by a higher incidence of cerebral haemorrhage (1.55%) than occurred with streptokinase (1.4%). Certainly TPA is much more expensive.

The benefits of early and appropriate use of any of the potential thrombolytic agents outweigh any potential advantages of any particular agent.

Gruppo Italiano per lo Studio della Sopravvivenza nell'Infarto Miocardico. GISSI-2: a factorial randomised trial of alteplase versus streptokinase and heparin versus no heparin among 12,490 patients with acute myocardial infarction. *Lancet* 1990; **336**(8707): 65–71.

ISIS-3 (Third International Study of Infarct Survival) Collaborative Group. ISIS-3: a randomised comparison of streptokinase vs tissue plasminogen activator vs anistreptase and of aspirin plus heparin vs aspirin alone among 41,299 cases of suspected acute myocardial infarction. *Lancet* 1992; **339**(8796): 753–70.

The GUSTO Investigators. An international randomized trial comparing four thrombolytic strategies for acute myocardial infarction. *N. Engl. J. Med.* 1993; **329**(10): 673–82.

8.9 You are caring for a ventilated patient who has been having large nasogastric aspirates. You are asked if it would be worthwhile to give him medication to enhance gastric emptying.

Is it likely to help, and what will you suggest?
Yes, there are data to support the concept that gastric emptying can be enhanced by pharmacological means in critically ill patients. Cisapride may be the most appropriate agent.

MINI-TUTORIAL

Metoclopramide blocks dopamine receptors (DA_1 and DA_2), but the prokinetic activity of metoclopramide appears to be mainly mediated by stimulation of intrinsic cholinergic nerves by activation of the 5-hydroxytryptamine type 4 receptor (5-HT4 receptor).

Cisapride actions include stimulation of the 5-HT4 receptor and direct increase of the release of acetylcholine from post-ganglionic nerve endings of the myenteric plexus (Fraser *et al.*, 1994).

Erythromycin has a motilin-like activity and has been shown to enhance gastric emptying and to induce large-amplitude antral pressure waves (Fraser *et al.*, 1992).

Addition of oral cisapride to an enteral feeding regimen has been shown to reverse the delayed gastric emptying which is characteristic in critically ill patients (Spapen *et al.*, 1995).

Fraser R, Horowitz M, Maddox A, Dent J. Postprandial antropyloroduodenal motility and gastric emptying in gastroparesis – effects of cisapride. *Gut* 1994; **35**: 172–8.

Fraser R, Shearer T, Fuller J, Horowitz M, Dent J. Intravenous erythromycin overcomes small intestinal feedback on antral, pyloric and duodenal motility. *Gastroenterology* 1992;**103**:114–19.

Spapen HD, Duinslaeger L, Diltoer M, Gillet R, Bossuyt A, Huyghens LP. Gastric emptying in critically ill patients is accelerated by adding cisapride to a standard enteral feeding protocol: results of a prospective, randomized, controlled trial. *Crit. Care Med.* 1995; **23**: 481–5.

8.10 You are on the ward round when the ICU specialist suggests that a patient would probably be a good candidate for 'immunonutrition'. He asks you to explain what 'immuno-nutrition' is.

What will you say?
Immunonutrition is the administration of feeds, supplemented with various nutrients, which beneficially alter the patient's immune status. Supplements include arginine, purine nucleotides and omega-3-poly-

unsaturated fatty acids. The basic rationale is that these supplements enhance immune function and consequently improve resistance to infection; however, modification of overactive inflammation and cytokine release may also be important.

Clinical trials suggest that the concept is useful and that use of 'immunomodulating' feeds (which generally contain several different supplements) can favourably influence outcome. Inevitably these special feeds cost significantly more than standard enteral feeds. The precise patient groups for whom 'immunonutrition' is best indicated have not yet been clearly defined.

Jolliet P and Pichard C. Immunonutrition in the critically ill. *Int. Care Med.* 1999; 25: 631–3.

8.11 A 23-year-old woman is admitted having taken a tricyclic overdose. She is hypotensive with a pulse rate of 116/minute and wide QRS complexes on the electrocardiogram. Her pH is 7.4 on arterial blood gas testing.

The Emergency registrar suggests that she should be given 8.4% sodium bicarbonate intravenously.

Do you agree?
Yes. The toxicity of tricyclic drugs appears to be reduced in the presence of alkalaemia.

MINI-TUTORIAL

In an observational study of 91 patients with tricyclic overdose hypotension resolved within 1 hour in 20 of 21 (96%) patients, QRS prolongation corrected in 39 of 49 (80%), and mental state improved in 40 of 85 (47%) following hypertonic sodium bicarbonate infusion. No complications associated with the administration of bicarbonate infusion were observed.

Hoffman JR, Votey SR, Bayer M, Silver L. Effect of hypertonic sodium bicarbonate in the treatment of moderate-to-severe cyclic antidepressant overdose. *Am. J. Emerg. Med.* 1993; **11**(4): 336–41.

9
Neurology

9.1 **A 17-year-old girl is admitted to the ICU with classical Guillain–Barré syndrome (ascending paralysis, delayed nerve conduction and raised CSF protein). The physician says she needs to receive plasmapheresis because this will reduce the chance that she will require ventilation and will help her to recover more quickly.**

(a) Do you agree with him?
Yes. There is evidence that plasmapheresis will be of benefit.

(b) If she is 'plasmapheresed', how much plasma should she have exchanged, how often and with what replacement fluid?
Looking at the studies which have supported the use of plasmapheresis, it is reasonable to perform four plasma exchanges, of two plasma volumes each, on alternate days. It is reasonable to use albumin in the replacement fluid rather than FFP.

MINI-TUTORIAL

In a multi-centre controlled trial in 220 patients with Guillain–Barré syndrome, plasma exchange ($n = 109$) was compared with standard treatment without plasma exchange ($n = 111$).

In the plasma exchange group 57 were assigned to receive albumin replacement while the other 52 received fresh frozen plasma (FFP).

The treatment group received four plasma exchanges, of two plasma volumes each, on alternate days.

Plasmapheresed patients had a reduction in the requirement for assisted ventilation, a decrease in time before beginning weaning from ventilation, reduced time to onset of motor recovery, and reduced time to walk.

No statistically significant difference was found between the group that received albumin and the group that received fresh frozen plasma (French Cooperative Group on Plasma Exchange in Guillain–Barré syndrome, 1987).

In a subsequent review of adverse effects in the study patients it was reported that FFP was associated with more adverse incidents than

---

albumin. Since the results with FFP did no better it was concluded by the authors that FFP should be abandoned as replacement fluid in plasma exchanges of Guillain–Barré syndrome patients (Bouget *et al.*, 1993).

Following acceptance of the efficacy of plasmapheresis in Guillain–Barré syndrome it became necessary to establish the relative value of intravenous immunoglobulin, which also appeared to be effective. This was determined in a further multi-centre trial.

Patients received either five plasma exchanges (each of 40 to 50 ml per kilogram of body weight) or five doses of intravenous immune globulin (0.4 g per kilogram per day).

Muscle strength improved by one grade or more in 34% of those treated with plasma exchange and 53% of those treated with immune globulin ($P < 0.05$). The median time to improvement by one grade was longer in patients treated with plasmapheresis (41 days) than with immune globulin therapy (27 days: $P = 0.05$). The immune globulin group had significantly fewer complications and less need for artificial ventilation. It was concluded that treatment with intravenous immune globulin is at least as effective as plasma exchange in the treatment of the acute Guillain–Barré syndrome, and may be superior (Van der Meche and Schmitz, 1992).

The role of high-dose steroids has also been evaluated in a large multi-centre, randomised, double-blind trial. 242 adult patients were randomised to receive intravenous methylprednisolone 500 mg (124 patients) or a placebo (118) daily for 5 days.

Some of these patients received plasma exchange, which was dependent on the practice of the recruiting hospital.

There was no significant difference in any outcome variable between patients treated with steroids and those given placebo. Consequently steroids are not recommended in the treatment of patients with Guillain–Barré syndrome (Guillain–Barré Syndrome Steroid Trial Group, 1993).

Bouget J, Chevret S, Chastang C, Raphael JC. Plasma exchange morbidity in Guillain–Barré syndrome: results from the French prospective, randomized, multicenter study: The French Cooperative Group. *Crit. Care Med.* 1993; **21**(5): 651–8.

French Cooperative Group on Plasma Exchange in Guillain–Barré syndrome. Efficiency of plasma exchange in Guillain–Barré syndrome: role of replacement fluids. *Ann. Neurol.* 1987; **22**(6): 753–61.

Guillain–Barré Syndrome Steroid Trial Group. Double-blind trial of intravenous methylprednisolone in Guillain–Barré syndrome. *Lancet* 1993; **341**(8845): 586–90.

Van der Meche FG, Schmitz PI. A randomized trial comparing intravenous immune globulin and plasma exchange in Guillain–Barré syndrome. Dutch Guillain–Barré Study Group. *N. Engl. J. Med.* 1992; **326**(17): 1123–9.

9.2 A 53-year-old man is intubated in the intensive care unit following resuscitation from an out-of-hospital cardiac arrest. It is now the third day after the arrest. He has no motor response to

pain but is breathing spontaneously. His pupils were unresponsive on admission but started reacting 14 hours afterwards.

The family are most concerned and ask you what you think the
chances of recovery are.

(a) What will you say?
Unfortunately there is minimal chance of a meaningful recovery in this
situation. Sadly, coma following hypoxic brain injury is a common
scenario in ICU following the introduction of out-of-hospital cardio-
pulmonary resuscitation, and an understanding of the predictors of
outcome is useful to assist in communication with families.

(b) Might any tests help to improve prediction of the outcome?
Yes. Testing of somatosensory evoked potentials are currently
considered the best determinant of outcome. MRI may be of value,
but this is yet to be clearly defined.

MINI-TUTORIAL

Few families seek for survival with severe disability (though for some this
is an acceptable goal). Consequently, those papers that deal with return
to independent function may be more useful than those which use
survival to assist decision making by families of patients with hypoxic
brain damage.

Outcome determination is difficult in the early period, but some
features are strongly associated with a poor outcome.

No patient with absent pupillary reflexes on initial examination ever
regained independent daily function in the report by Levy *et al.* (1985). In
the same report most patients with poor outcome were identified within
24 hours following presentation. Of patients with motor responses that
were worse than localising, or spontaneous eye movements that were
neither orienting nor roving conjugate, 93% failed to return to independent function (Levy *et al.*, 1985)

Prognosis can be predicted with more certainty at 72 hours when
absence of reflexes assumes more significance and by which time neurological testing can also be used to improve the prediction of outcome.

Results from neurological examination, electroencephalogram
(EEG), or somatosensory evoked potentials (SSEP) have been evaluated with respect to their relationship to poor outcome – (defined as
death or survival in a vegetative state) in a review of 33 studies by
Zandbergen *et al.* (1998).

From these studies three variables were found to have a specificity of
100% (i.e. were never associated with an outcome better than death or
persistent vegetative state). These were:

- absence of pupillary light reflexes on day 3
- absent motor response to pain on day 3
- bilateral absence of early cortical SSEP within the first week.

In addition, EEG recordings with an isoelectric or burst-suppression pattern had a specificity of 100% in five of six studies where EEG findings were reported.

Since evoked potentials (SSEP) are also the least susceptible to metabolic changes and drugs, it was concluded that recording of SSEP is the most useful method to predict poor outcome.

Levy DE, Caronna JJ, Singer BH, Lapinski RH, Frydman H, Plum F. Predicting outcome from hypoxic-ischemic coma. *JAMA* 1985; **253**(10): 1420–6.

Zandbergen EG, de Haan RJ, Stoutenbeek CP, Koelman JH, Hijdra A. Systematic review of early prediction of poor outcome in anoxic-ischaemic coma. *Lancet* 1998; **352**(9143): 1808–12.

9.3 A 65-year-old man has a cardiac arrest at home. He receives adequate CPR by his relatives and is cardioverted to sinus rhythm within 15 minutes with blood pressure of 120/80 mmHg. He remains intubated and ventilated and has an extensor response to pain. Six hours later his neurological status is unchanged and he begins to have continuous myoclonic seizures. His family are at the bedside and ask you what the fitting means.

What is the implication of the seizures?

Seizures occur in some form in approximately one third of patients with post-hypoxic encephalopathy. Isolated seizures are not associated with a poorer prognosis.

Status epilepticus is a poor prognostic sign. Myoclonic status epilepticus (MSE) is the most common form of status epilepticus seen following cerebral hypoxia, and has the poorest prognosis.

MINI-TUTORIAL

MSE can be very difficult to control with standard benzodiazepines, barbiturates and phenytoin. Enormous doses may be required (Krumholz *et al.*, 1988).

Wijdicks *et al.* (1994) reported on 107 patients who remained comatose after cardiac resuscitation. They found that myoclonus status occurs relatively commonly (37%). All patients with myoclonus status died. They concluded that myoclonus status in post-anoxic coma is indicative of devastating cerebral damage.

Krumholz A, Stern BJ, Weiss H. Outcome from coma after cardiopulmonary resuscitation: Relation to seizures and myoclonus. *Neurology* 1988; **38**: 401–5.
Wijdicks EF, Parisi JE, Sharbrough FW. Prognostic value of myoclonus status in comatose survivors of cardiac arrest. *Ann. Neurol.* 1994; **35**(2): 239–43.

9.4 You are asked to review a 15-year-old boy who is on the surgical ward with a tracheostomy who has developed a pneumonia. He has a diagnosis of persistent vegetative state (PVS) following a head injury 6 weeks before. It appears that he is going into respiratory failure and requires ventilation. Before accepting further 'high-tech' support the boy's parents wish to know what chance there is that their son might improve.

(a) What will you tell them?
There is a chance that he might improve (up to 50%) but probably less than a 20% chance that he could eventually become independent. Had he been in PVS for longer than 12 months then the chance of improvement would be minimal.

(b) Might any tests assist you to predict his chance of recovery?
Cerebral magnetic resonance imaging (MRI) performed between 6 weeks and 8 weeks after injury has been reported to improve prediction of outcome.

MINI-TUTORIAL

Vegetative state is a state where the patient shows no evidence of awareness of self or environment but does exhibit cycles of sleep and wakefulness. Persistent vegetative state (PVS) is a vegetative state that continues for at least one month.

The potential for improvement depends upon aetiology and age (younger patients or those with traumatic aetiology have potentially more chance of recovery than is the case with older patients or following anoxic brain injury). Recovery of consciousness from a post-traumatic persistent vegetative state is unlikely after 12 months in both adults and children. Recovery from a non-traumatic persistent vegetative state after three months is exceedingly rare in both adults and children.

It is well recognised that children have a much better possibility of improvement from PVS than do adults. In a large study of patients with PVS, Hendl and Laub (1996) observed that a significant number changed from PVS: 84% of the patients with traumatic brain injury group and 55% of the hypoxic brain injury patients.

Although the children improved, few became independent in everyday life (16% of patients with traumatic aetiology), particularly following hypoxic brain injury (4% became independent).

Since delayed improvement is possible, particularly in post-traumatic vegetative state, it would be most useful to be able to predict patients who might recover. This has not been possible, but there is a suggestion that cerebral magnetic resonance imaging (MRI) might be useful.

The predictive value of cerebral magnetic resonance imaging (MRI) performed between 6 weeks and 8 weeks after injury has been evaluated in 80 adult patients in post-traumatic vegetative state (Kampfl et al., 1998).

In the subsequent 12 months, 38 patients had improved while 42 patients had not.

Patients who did not improve had a significantly higher frequency of corpus callosum, corona radiata, and dorsolateral brainstem injuries than did patients who did improve.

Heindl UT, Laub MC. Outcome of persistent vegetative state following hypoxic or traumatic brain injury in children and adolescents. *Neuropediatrics* 1996; **27**(2): 94–100.
Kampfl A *et al.* Prediction of recovery from post-traumatic vegetative state with cerebral magnetic-resonance imaging. *Lancet* 1998; **351**(9118): 1763–7.
The Multi-Society Task Force on PVS. Medical aspects of the persistent vegetative state (1). *N. Engl. J. Med.* 1994; **330**(21): 1499–508.

9.5 You are asked to admit a 45-year-old woman who is apnoeic, completely unresponsive to pain and has fixed dilated pupils. She was found at home deeply cyanosed and hypotensive with minimal respiratory effort. She appears to have taken a massive propranolol overdose. Both the ambulance officers and the medical resident think she has suffered significant cerebral hypoxia. The medical resident asks if you think she could be an organ donor.

What will you say?
Somebody who is certified brain dead may be considered for organ donation. This patient does not satisfy the criteria for brain death since the precondition of 'absence of drug intoxication' is not satisfied. Describing a patient as brain dead or talking about organ donation before formal confirmation is most inappropriate and may cause considerable problems especially if the relatives are involved ('the doctor said she was brain dead and now she is going home'). If relatives raise the issue you should clearly state that the patient is not

brain dead (since this state occurs when brain death testing is completed), although the patient may indeed become brain dead. You cannot be criticised for such a statement. Patients with large drug overdoses are often completely unresponsive and have fixed dilated pupils; however, they usually recover rapidly and without obvious deficit.

MINI-TUTORIAL

Essential prerequisites for brain death testing

- A cause of brain injury leading to a state of deep coma and apnoea must be clear and unequivocal.
- There must be no influence of sedative or muscle relaxant drugs.
- There must be no metabolic or endocrine cause for coma.
- Significant hypothermia must not be present.
- The systolic pressure should be adequate to maintain cerebral function (if present) (> 80 mmHg).

Clinical testing

- No pupil response to light.
- No corneal reflex.
- No response to pain in the distribution of the trigeminal nerve (V).
- No facial (VII) response to pain in any somatic area.
- No cough or gag response.
- No nystagmus in response to cold water irrigation of the ears.
- No respiratory activity during observed apnoea with oxygen insufflation adequate to raise the $P_a\text{CO}_2$ to 60 mmHg (8 kPa).

Where pre-conditions cannot be met

- Four vessel angiography (both carotids and both vertebral arteries) with demonstration of absence of flow within the skull from any of the vessels will confirm brain death.

Diagnosis of brain death. Conference of Medical Royal Colleges and their Faculties in the United Kingdom. *Br. Med. J.* 1976 Nov 13; **2**(6045): 1187–8.
Diagnosis of brain death. *Lancet* 1976 Nov 13; **2**(7994): 1069–70.

9.6 During apnoea testing to confirm brain death in a 23-year-old man he is seen to partially sit up by bending forward at the hips and his arms flex at the elbows and leave the bed. There is great consternation among those witnessing this.

What does this movement mean?

This is a spinal reflex. This movement is termed the 'Lazarus sign'. It is well recognised to occur in brain dead patients, but is fortunately rare.

MINI-TUTORIAL

It is important to recognise that spinal mediated movement may occur, since this is very disturbing to witness. Movement, should it occur, is most likely following ventilator disconnection when the spinal cord becomes hypoxic and acidotic. If it happens at one disconnection it is likely to recur subsequently; conversely if it does not happen during the first test it is unlikely to occur during later tests.

Similarly, reflex hypertension and tachycardia is well recognised in response to surgical stress in organ donors; such changes should not throw doubt on a properly performed diagnosis of brain death.

Fitzgerald RD, Dechtyar I, Templ E, Fridrich P, Lackner FX. Cardiovascular and catecholamine response to surgery in brain-dead organ donors. *Anaesthesia* 1995; **50**(5): 388–92.

Heytens L, Verlooy J, Gheuens J, Bossaert L. Lazarus sign and extensor posturing in a brain-dead patient – Case report. *J. Neurosurg.* 1989; **71**(3): 449–51.

10

Pulmonary artery catheter

10.1 You are caring for a 74-year-old man with a long history of chronic obstructive airways disease and known pulmonary hypertension. He is known to have had myocardial infarctions in the past. He is now very septic and hypotensive.

There is debate about the wisdom of using his CVP to manage his fluid balance.

What do you think?

There is certainly a strong feeling that pulmonary artery catheters do not need to be used as frequently as they are at present. However, the situation described (COAD, pulmonary hypertension, myocardial infarction and severe illness) is just that where the value of the CVP poorly predicts the left-sided pressures.

MINI-TUTORIAL

CVP generally provides a good estimate of left atrial pressure in patients with normal cardio-pulmonary function. However, in critically ill patients the right and left ventricles may have significant differences in pre-load, compliance, and stroke volume and consequently the CVP may poorly predict left ventricular filling pressure. In patients with chronic obstructive airways disease, especially in those with cardiac dysfunction as a result of chronic pulmonary hypertension, the CVP and wedge pressure show poor correlation.

Toussaint GP, Burgess JH, Hampson LG. Central venous pressure and pulmonary wedge pressure in critical surgical illness: a comparison. *Arch. Surg.* 1974; **109**: 265–9.

10.2 There is discussion on the ward round about the value of pulmonary artery catheterisation in a patient with sepsis and previous myocardial infarction. An ICU registrar states that 'there is conclusive evidence that pulmonary artery catheterisation helps to direct treatment and improves outcome in critically ill patients'.

Is he correct?

Sadly not. It may help to direct therapy, but a beneficial impact on outcome has not been proved. Indeed, on current evidence there is a suggestion that patients treated with a pulmonary artery catheter might do worse than those managed without it.

MINI-TUTORIAL

The impact of the use of a pulmonary artery catheter during the first 24 h of care in the ICU on subsequent survival has been evaluated in a large prospective cohort study. Data from a total of 5735 critically ill adult patients were examined and 2016 pairs were matched (one with a PA catheter and one without). The investigators found an *increased* mortality in patients in whom a PA catheter was used (Connors *et al.*, 1996).

The matching was difficult and it remains possible that the group in which physicians used PA catheters were sicker. The study provided no information as to the cause of death, thus making it difficult to assess how a PA catheter inserted on the first day in the ICU impacts on death on day 5, day 30 or after 6 months (the observation points).

This study has caused some consternation, with some authors advocating that pulmonary artery catheter use should be severely restricted until definitive proof of benefit in specific patient groups is demonstrated. The situation is probably a condemnation of the widespread adoption of technology without careful evaluation. The study did not investigate what actions were taken in response to the data (obviously monitoring data must be appropriately acted upon otherwise no outcome benefit can result). Most practitioners of intensive care feel that there is a valuable role for pulmonary artery catheterisation (exactly how much and in which patients is debatable), but currently the evidence base is not supportive.

Connors AF, Jr, Speroff T, Dawson NV *et al.* The effectiveness of right heart catheterization in the initial care of critically ill patients: SUPPORT Investigators. *JAMA* 1996; **276**: 889–97.

10.3 You are asked to put in a pulmonary artery catheter in the early hours of the morning. Before you start the ICU specialist asks you (in order to check how aware you are of the issues) which approaches are best for pulmonary arterial catheterisation, and also asks what you need to do before inserting the catheter.

What will you say?

Since the catheter inserts most easily when the curve at the tip does not require rotation the easiest (and therefore preferred) approaches are via the right internal jugular vein or the left subclavian vein) (Fig. 10.1).

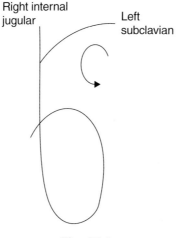

Right internal jugular

Left subclavian

Fig. 10.1

MINI-TUTORIAL

When observing pressure changes so as to position a pulmonary artery catheter, it is essential that the pressure monitoring is operating correctly before the catheter is inserted and that the operator is aware of the expected pressure changes as the catheter passes through the heart and pulmonary artery. If the transducer is not correctly attached and zeroed, or the tubing is not properly flushed, then you have little chance of successfully placing the catheter.

10.4 When ready to insert the pulmonary artery catheter you move the tip up and down rapidly and observe the trace on the screen. The trace looks like Fig. 10.2.

Fig. 10.2

(a) What might be the problem?

After priming the catheter and checking the balloon, but before beginning to insert the catheter, it is important to move the tip up and down briskly and to determine that this is rapidly and accurately reflected on the displayed PA trace. Reasons why no response is seen include failure to connect the cable to the transducer, selection of the wrong waveform on the monitor, turned off three-way taps to the catheter or failure to zero the transducer correctly.

Following connection of the cable and zeroing the trace looks like Fig. 10.3 when the tip is moved up and down rapidly.

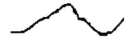

Fig. 10.3

(b) What is the problem now?

The pressure response is damped (it rises slowly and falls slowly). In this situation the usual cause is a bubble in the tubing (this air compresses when pressurised and absorbs the pressure). Flush the system well (including knocking or shaking the system if bubbles prove difficult to dislodge).

Following flushing the trace looks like Fig. 10.4 when the tip is moved up and down rapidly.

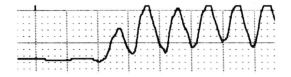

Fig. 10.4

(c) What do you think now?

Now it is fine! You can now proceed to insert it. This is an important point: if you proceed to try to insert the catheter before you check this you will not know where you are and will fail.

MINI-TUTORIAL

When the catheter is inserted through the introducer sheath and the balloon is beyond the end of the sheath and in the superior vena cava the balloon is inflated with air. The catheter then floats through the right atrium and ventricle, through the pulmonary outflow tract, and into the pulmonary artery. Finally, it wedges in the distal pulmonary artery.

When correctly positioned the distal lumen (at the tip) is in the pulmonary artery and the proximal lumen is in the right atrium.

10.5 There is some discussion about a patient's fluid requirements. The surgical registrar insists that the patient is 'underfilled'. To facilitate the discussion a trace is recorded for you to check the wedge pressure (Fig. 10.5).

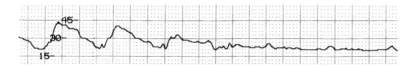

Fig. 10.5

What value is the wedge pressure?
The wedge pressure is approximately 20 mmHg (assuming the transducer is correctly zeroed). This supports the contention that the patient has adequate or excessive intravascular volume.

MINI-TUTORIAL

On a good pulmonary artery wedge pressure, 'a', 'c' and 'v' waves can be identified. The 'a' and 'v' waves are generally of similar magnitude in most patients and a mean end expiratory pulmonary wedge pressure (generally referred to as the 'wedge pressure') gives a good reflection of the left atrial filling pressure.

In patients with marked mitral regurgitation there is a large 'v' wave on the pulmonary wedge pressure trace. The large 'v' wave is caused by the systolic regurgitant flow.

10.6 You are asked to look at the pulmonary artery catheter trace of Fig. 10.6. There is some concern that it is not properly wedging; if it is wedged, at what point on the trace should the wedge pressure be read?

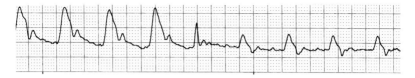

Fig. 10.6

What do you think?

The trace shows satisfactory wedging, but there are prominent 'v' waves on the wedged trace. These 'v' waves are seen in cases of mitral regurgitation. Where large 'v' waves are present on the wedge trace, an estimate of the left ventricular end diastolic pressure is best determined from the crest of the 'a' wave in patients in sinus rhythm. In patients in atrial fibrillation the left ventricular end diastolic pressure is taken from the base of the waveform (just before the upstroke of the 'v' wave).

MINI-TUTORIAL

Sometimes in cases of severe mitral regurgitation it can be difficult to differentiate the pulmonary arterial pressure trace from that after wedging due to the large 'v' waves still present on the trace. The 'v' wave occurs later in the cardiac cycle than does the pulmonary arterial systolic wave, which is seen together with the 'v' wave when the balloon is deflated and the catheter is not wedged (only the 'v' wave is seen when the catheter is wedged).

10.7 You are asked to look at the pulmonary artery catheter of a 72-year-old man who has had an aortic valve replacement. It is thought that the balloon 'won't wedge'.

One hour earlier the trace looked like Fig. 10.7:

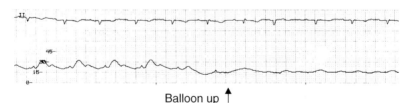

Balloon up ↑

Fig. 10.7

Now it looks like Fig. 10.8:

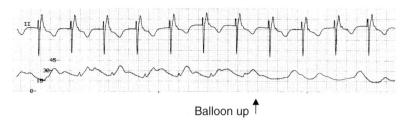

Balloon up ↑

Fig. 10.8

What do you think is going on?
In Fig. 10.7 the patient is in sinus rhythm. The wedge trace is normal without evidence of prominent 'v' waves.

Fig. 10.8 has altered from a characteristic arterial trace to one with only one wave per cycle once the balloon is inflated. This is a marked 'v' wave on the wedge trace and indicates that the patient has developed significant mitral regurgitation. The ECG trace has also altered and is characteristic of ventricular paced rhythm. The ventricular pacing is causing discoordinate ventricular contraction with the generation of significant mitral regurgitation. Ventricular pacing is often associated with reduced cardiac output (vs. sinus rhythm). This can be due to loss of atrial kick and the induction of mitral regurgitation.

10.8 A 63-year-old woman is ventilated for respiratory failure complicating left ventricular failure. She is on SIMV with 600 ml tidal volume and is taking no spontaneous breaths. A pulmonary artery catheter is *in situ*. See Fig. 10.9.

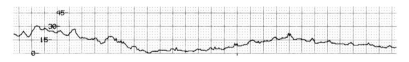

Fig. 10.9

What is the wedge pressure?
2 mmHg.

MINI-TUTORIAL

PAWP measurements are best obtained when the patient is supine and at end expiration, when pleural pressure is closest to zero.

 Where there is a notable respiratory swing the upper part of the curve is expiration in spontaneously breathing patients (since there is negative pressure during inspiration). Conversely the lower part of the curve corresponds with expiration in patients on intermittent positive pressure ventilation (since there is positive pressure during inspiration).

10.9 A 65-year-old man with asthma and myocardial infarction has a pulmonary artery catheter inserted to evaluate whether his dyspnoea is due to left ventricular failure or to his asthma. See Fig. 10.10.

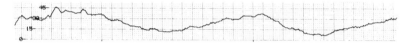

Fig. 10.10

What do you think his wedge pressure is?
Accurate measurement is very difficult in patients with huge respiratory swings.

 Patients with respiratory distress and laboured breathing have deep inspiratory troughs and high expiratory peaks of intra-thoracic pressure (Fig. 10.11). These are reflected in the pulmonary artery wedge pressure trace, which shows significant swings with respiration. These large variations make determination of the Paw difficult. Observation of the patient to establish the precise point between exhalation and inspiration (end exhalation) and matching this with the pressure trace may help. Alternatively, in appropriate patients in whom it is indicated, sedation and ventilation with paralysis will simplify interpretation of the pressure trace. In the intensive care setting most patients with uninterpretable traces due to respiratory variation have such severe respiratory distress that they require intubation anyway.

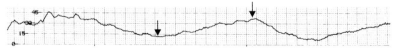

Large inspiratory negative pressure   Large expiratory positive pressure

Fig. 10.11

MINI-TUTORIAL

The pulmonary artery diastolic (Pad) pressure is generally 1–4 mm above the left atrial pressure. When the catheter cannot be wedged (e.g. because of balloon rupture) the Pad can usually be used as a substitute estimate of left atrial pressure. However, increased pulmonary vascular resistance will increase the gradient between the PADP and PAWP. (Where there are prior measurements of Pad, Paw and CVP, the relationship between these can be observed and this can be taken into account for ongoing interpretation).

10.10 The trace in Fig. 10.12 is obtained from a patient following the pulmonary artery catheter being advanced because it would not 'wedge'. The top trace is the CVP (proximal lumen) and the lower the pulmonary artery pressure (distal, tip lumen).

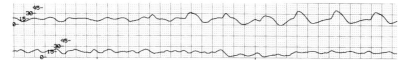

Fig. 10.12

What do you think has caused the change to the CVP trace?
The CVP trace is showing a right ventricular pressure pattern.

The catheter has been advanced too far and the proximal (CVP) lumen is now in the right ventricle. If the proximal lumen is in the right ventricle then the tip must be too far into the pulmonary artery or the catheter must be looped in the ventricle. In either case it should be withdrawn.

10.11 You are told that there is difficulty getting a good pulmonary artery wedge trace. On inflation of the balloon the trace looks like Fig. 10.13:

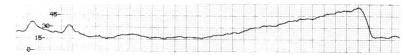

Fig. 10.13

(a) What is happening?
This is known as 'over wedging'. It occurs when the catheter is in too far and the balloon is distending a small artery. After initially falling the pressure goes up progressively as the balloon is inflated. The pressure here rises *above* the PA systolic, which is not possible (or blood would be flowing backwards through the lungs!). NEVER continue to inflate the balloon if the trace rises above the PA systolic.

(b) What needs to be done?
STOP inflating the balloon! – or the artery will rupture. The tip of the catheter is too far into the pulmonary vessels in a small branch. The catheter needs to be pulled back and the balloon should then be cautiously reinflated to ensure that a normal trace is produced at full inflation of the balloon.

Later you are told that the catheter 'won't wedge' and air isn't coming back into the syringe after inflating the balloon. It is suggested that a wedge trace might be obtained if a bigger syringe is used to inflate the balloon.

(c) What do you think?
No! The air must be able to be aspirated (or move spontaneously) back into the syringe. Where this does not occur it is likely that the balloon has ruptured. This is supported by the failure to wedge (often the hole is small, the balloon still inflates but then deflates before the wedge can be measured). Repeatedly injecting air into the pulmonary circulation is bad for the patient, so suggesting injecting more is frightening. Check the balloon once and stop using it if balloon rupture is confirmed.

10.12 A man with a ruptured mitral valve who is being supported on an intra-aortic balloon pump does not appear to be augmenting well. You are asked if you think the timing is the problem.

What are your goals when adjusting the timing of intra-aortic balloon inflation?
The balloon should be inflated just after the closure of the aortic valve (indicated on the pressure wave form by the dichrotic notch) and should be deflated before the aortic valve reopens (indicated on the pressure wave form by the rapid ascent of blood pressure).

MINI-TUTORIAL

Inflating too early while the aortic valve is still open will increase the left ventricular workload. Inflating late results in reduced augmentation (diastolic aortic root pressure rises less) and consequently left ventricular coronary perfusion (which occurs during diastole) is not enhanced.

Deflation should occur just prior to systole. Ideally, deflation is adjusted to achieve the lowest aortic pressure just prior to systole. Deflating the balloon too early reduces the time that increased diastolic pressure augments coronary perfusion, while deflating too late results in systolic ejection of blood being impeded by the inflated balloon, with an unnecessary increase in left ventricular work.

10.13 On a ward round you overhear a surgical registrar explaining to a student that helium is used to drive the balloon of the intra-aortic balloon pump (IABP) because it is very soluble in blood. Consequently, should balloon rupture occur it is less likely to cause gas embolism than other gases, such as carbon dioxide.

Is this the reason helium is used?
No. Helium is poorly soluble in blood and gas embolism is a risk.

Helium is used because its low density permits the high gas velocities necessary at elevated heart rates to inflate and deflate the balloon within one cardiac cycle. Gases such as carbon dioxide or oxygen do not flow quickly enough for this purpose.

10.14 A 63-year-old man who had a mitral valve replacement (St Jude, mechanical valve) 9 days ago is readmitted to the ICU. He has made slow progress since his operation and has become acutely hypotensive and dyspnoeic on the general ward. The trace in Fig. 10.14 is observed on his monitor immediately after ICU admission. The ICU specialist is at home (it is 2 a.m.) and asks you what you think is going on.

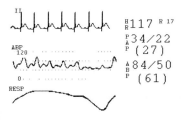

Fig. 10.14

What will you say?
He is in sinus tachycardia with some concave ST elevation (probably non-specific following recent cardiac surgery, but ischaemia is possible). The arterial pressure shows a very profound drop in time with respiratory inhalation. This is 'pulsus paradoxus'. It suggests cardiac tamponade (although pulsus paradoxus can also occur in severe asthma, but not usually of this magnitude), which is a reasonable diagnosis on clinical grounds in a man on warfarin following recent surgery. The presence of a significant volume of fluid blood in the pericardium is confirmed by transthoracic echocardiography, and following drainage he is much improved.

10.15 You are treating a patient who is hypotensive with a low pulmonary artery wedge pressure (PAWP) who requires intravascular filling. There is some discussion about the choice of fluid. One ICU registrar tells you that there is evidence that colloids increase mortality, while the other says that there is no such evidence and that the choice of either colloid or crystalloid is valid.

Who is correct?
The controversy about the optimal fluid for use in resuscitation and intravascular fluid expansion in critically ill patients has been ongoing for many years. There is currently no clear answer. Recent reviews have come to different conclusions: one that colloid is harmful and should not be used, the other that there is no difference in outcome whichever is used. Both registrars are expressing opinions for which there is support. Given the controversy and lack of definitive studies, it might be honest not to ferociously advocate either view.

MINI-TUTORIAL

Following a meta-analysis of randomised trials of crystalloid or colloid administration to critically ill patients, one group of reviewers concluded that the data suggest that mortality is increased in patients resuscitated with colloid (Schierhout *et al.*, 1998). Another group, which essentially addressed the same question and reviewed similar studies, concluded that there is no apparent difference in pulmonary oedema, mortality or length of stay in ICU whether patients are given colloid or crystalloid for resuscitation (Choi *et al.*, 1999).

Crystalloids cost less than colloids and do not cause anaphylaxis. However, the infusion of crystalloids results in reduction of oncotic pressure, which may predispose to pulmonary and peripheral tissue oedema. The rapid distribution of crystalloid through the extra-cellular fluid requires that more volume of crystalloid be administered to achieve the filling pressure (CVP or PAWP) goals than is the case for colloids.

Very few studies have shown any specific benefit (observing any potentially useful end point) when colloids have been used. Consequently, while it may be concluded that colloid administration may not be harmful, it is difficult with the available evidence to define clinical situations where colloids are indicated.

Synthetic colloids (e.g. Haemaccel) have not been included in these reviews (because they were not included in the studies), and consequently the conclusions of these reviews cannot be used with respect to these agents.

Choi P, Yip G, Quinonez L, Cook D. Crystalloids vs colloids in fluid resuscitation: A systematic review. *Crit. Care Med.* 1999; **27**: 200–10.

Schierhout G, Roberts I. Fluid resuscitation with colloid or crystalloid solutions in critically ill patients: A systematic review of randomised trials. *BMJ* 1998; 316: 961–4.

10.16 You are managing a 63-year-old man who has severe peritonitis which has complicated a traumatic rupture of the caecum (which was not diagnosed until two days after injury). He currently has a cardiac index of 4.1 l/min/m^2, his saturation is 95% and his haemoglobin is 99 g/l. The anaesthetic registrar tells you that you need to increase his oxygen delivery.

(a) Why is he suggesting this?
There was a period in intensive care practice when 'supranormal' oxygen delivery was advocated and practised in many units.

Oxygen delivery (DO$_2$) is calculated as:

Oxygen carrying capacity of haemoglobin (ml/g Hb) × Hb (in g/dl) × $S_{a}O_2$/100 × CI/100

(Oxygen carrying capacity of haemoglobin = 1.39 ml/g Hb.)

In this case DO$_2$ = 1.39 × 9.9 × 0.95 × 41 = 536 ml/min/m^2. 'Supranormal' oxygen delivery goal would be > 650 ml/min/m^2.

(b) What will you do?
Change nothing.

Firstly, when instructed to do things by 'visitors' from outside ICU report their 'requests and suggestions' to the senior staff in ICU for consideration.

In this specific instance use of 'supranormal' oxygen delivery goals is no longer advocated (see below).

MINI-TUTORIAL

Normally oxygen consumption (VO_2) remains relatively constant over a wide range of rates of oxygen delivery (DO_2), since oxygen extraction increases as oxygen delivery decreases. However, oxygen consumption becomes dependent on DO_2 below 5–10 ml/kg per min, since extraction becomes maximal.

It has been reported that oxygen consumption increases as oxygen delivery is increased in critically ill patients with sepsis or ARDS. This increased oxygen consumption has been reported to continue up to high levels of oxygen delivery (> 20 ml/kg per min)(Mohensifar *et al.*, 1983). It was consequently advocated that 'supranormal' DO_2 and haemodynamic values should be therapeutic goals in these patients. Using this approach, lower mortality figures have been reported (Shoemaker *et al.*, 1993; Tuschmidt *et al.*, 1992).

However, this 'pathological supply dependence' concept has fallen into disrepute. In the earlier studies, VO_2 was calculated rather than measured, and a resultant VO_2/DO_2 relationship was possible from mathematical coupling (e.g. cardiac output features in both the calculation of VO_2 and DO_2, so increasing the cardiac output will result in a rise in both, although VO_2 may not actually increase) (Hanique *et al.*, 1994). More recent studies in which VO_2 is directly measured have not shown a pathological VO_2/DO_2 relationship nor better patient outcome with 'supranormal' therapy (Heyland *et al.*, 1996; Alia *et al.*, 1999).

Currently supranormal oxygen delivery goals are not advocated in critically ill patients.

Alia I, Esteban A, Gordo F, Lorente JA, Diaz C, Rodriguez JA, Frutos F. A randomized and controlled trial of the effect of treatment aimed at maximizing oxygen delivery in patients with severe sepsis or septic shock. *Chest* 1999; **115**(2): 453–61.

Hanique G, Dugernier T, Laterre PF, Dougnac A, Roeseler J, Reynaert MS. Significance of pathologic oxygen supply dependence in critically ill patients: comparison between measured and calculated methods. *Int. Care Med.* 1994; **20**: 12–18.

Heyland DK, Cook DJ, King D, Kernerman P, Brun-Buisson C. Maximizing oxygen delivery in critically ill patients: a methodologic appraisal of the evidence. *Crit. Care Med.* 1996; **24**(3): 517–24.

Mohensifar Z, Goldbach P, Tashkin DP *et al.* Relationship between O_2 delivery and O_2 consumption in the adult respiratory distress syndrome. *Chest* 1983; **84**: 267–71.

Shoemaker WC, Appel PL, Kram HB. Hemodynamic and oxygen transport responses in survivors and nonsurvivors of high-risk surgery. *Crit. Care Med.* 1993; **21**: 977–90.

Tuschmidt J, Fired J, Astiz M, Rackow E. Elevation of cardiac output and oxygen delivery improves outcome in septic shock. *Chest* 1992; **102**: 216–20.

10.17 You have just increased the noradrenaline dose in a patient with sepsis who has a low blood pressure and low vascular resistance. The surgeon who operated on him suggests that the noradrenaline 'is probably making his guts ischaemic'. He says that you can monitor the pH of the gastric fluid to determine whether the stomach is getting ischaemic.

Is he correct about this monitoring?
No. It has been suggested that monitoring of the gastric intramucosal pH (termed pHi) by monitoring of intragastric CO_2 levels can detect gastric ischaemia. This has nothing to do with the pH of the fluid secreted into the stomach.

MINI-TUTORIAL

Gut intraluminal P_{CO_2} levels are recognised to rise promptly (< 1 minute) and significantly in response to reductions in gut perfusion (Morgan *et al.*, 1997). It is suggested that this CO_2 rise results from reaction of hydrogen ions produced in the ischaemic mucosa with bicarbonate in the interstitial fluid ($H^+ + HCO_3^- = CO_2 + H_2O$). The CO_2 diffuses into the bowel lumen where it can be measured directly (by CO_2 electrode) or, more often, after equilibration with air or saline in a gas-permeable silicone balloon in the bowel.

Equilibration with saline is slow (and some blood gas machines give inaccurate readings for P_{CO_2} in saline) while equilibration with air is more rapid.

The gastric intramucosal pH (pHi) is calculated from a modified Henderson–Hasselbalch equation using the arterial HCO_3^- and the P_{CO_2} from the gastric tonometer (the pHi has nothing to do with the gastric pH or secretion of acid from the stomach in the process of digestion).

Interpretation of pHi is complicated by the fact that a low HCO_3^- due to systemic acidosis will lead to a low result for pHi, even though gut perfusion is normal. Equally a high arterial P_{CO_2} due to respiratory failure (or permissive hypercapnia) will equilibrate with intraluminal gas and give a low pHi result (independently of gut perfusion). Consideration of the difference between intraluminal and arterial P_{CO_2} avoids the problems outlined above.

Further errors can be introduced by generation of CO_2 from the reaction of refluxing bicarbonate rich pancreatic secretion into the stomach where reaction with stomach acid liberates CO_2 (avoided by the use of ranitidine to block gastric acid production). The use of effervescent soluble drugs will markedly raise gastric CO_2 levels.

Despite early enthusiasm for a method to monitor gut perfusion the problems associated with the technique and the observed difficulty of improving abnormal results by treatment has not encouraged wide-spread use of the technique.

Morgan TJ, Venkatesh B, Endre ZH. Continuous measurement of gut luminal $P_a CO_2$ in the rat: responses to transient episodes of graded aortic hypotension *Crit. Care Med.* 1997; **25**(9): 1575–8.
Russell JA. Gastric tonometry: does it work? *Int. Care Med.* 1997; **23**(1): 3–6.

10.18 An obese 39-year-old woman is admitted urgently to ICU. She earlier suffered a collapse on the medical ward where she had been admitted with a diagnosis of pleurisy. A ventilation/perfusion scan has been done and is highly suggestive of multiple pulmonary emboli. On admission she is peripherally shut down with a blood pressure of 75/45 and a heart rate of 136/min.

There is a discussion about the role of thrombolyis in this lady. The medical registrar says that in her opinion thrombolysis is clearly indicated.

What do you think?
She is correct. This patient is haemodynamically unstable and both evidence and practice guidelines support thrombolysis.

Thrombolysis offers a number of potential advantages in the treatment of patients with pulmonary thrombo-embolism:

- More rapid pulmonary clot lysis will result in more rapid restoration of pulmonary perfusion and resolution of pulmonary hypertension and right heart dysfunction.
- More rapid venous clot lysis will reduce the incidence of recurrent pulmonary embolism.
- More rapid pulmonary clot resolution and reduction of recurrent embolism should reduce the incidence of chronic pulmonary vascular obstruction with resultant pulmonary hypertension.

MINI-TUTORIAL

Thrombolytic therapy results in more rapid clot resolution than treatment with heparin alone and appears to improve prognosis in patients with shock due to massive pulmonary embolism. In haemodynamically stable patients thrombolysis has not been shown to reduce mortality or recurrent embolism. However, it appears that a subset of patients who have normal systemic arterial blood pressure but are shown to have a dilated dysfunctional right ventricle on investigation may have reduced mortality when treated with thrombolysis.

Thrombolysis may improve the haemodynamic response to exercise in long-term survivors.

A two-hour regimen of thrombolysis is advocated, as this appears to result in more rapid clot resolution than do more prolonged infusions.

Major haemorrhage (i.e. that causing intra-cranial haemorrhage or bleeding requiring surgery or transfusion) occurs in 12% of patients given thrombolysis for pulmonary embolism and 1.8% of those given heparin alone. Intra-cranial haemorrhage occurs in 1.2% of patients given thrombolytics, but in none treated only with heparin.

Arcasoy SM, Kreit JW. Thrombolytic therapy of pulmonary embolism. A comprehensive review of current evidence. *Chest* 1999;**115**: 1695–707.

11

ECG strips

11.1 You are called urgently to review a 73-year-old man who has become hypotensive and dyspnoeic. He had a pneumonectomy two days ago and has subsequently had some trouble with sputum retention. An ECG strip is available for you to look at (Fig. 11.1):

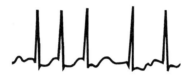

Fig. 11.1

(a) What does the rhythm strip show?
Rapid atrial fibrillation.

(b) What will you suggest needs to be done?
This patient would benefit from reverting to sinus rhythm. If he is severely compromised DC cardioversion is indicated; otherwise rate control and increased tendency to revert can be achieved by amiodarone.

11.2 An 85-year-old woman is admitted from a medical ward with hypotension. The intern admitting her notes that her pulse rate is slow and runs off a rhythm strip (Fig. 11.2):

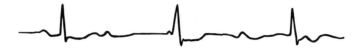

Fig. 11.2

(a) What does the rhythm strip show?
Complete heart block.

(b) What will you suggest needs to be done?
She requires transvenous pacing. Temporarily the rate can be increased by isoprenaline.

11.3 A 65-year-old man with cardiomyopathy is admitted to ICU for treatment of acute pulmonary oedema. The student nurse who escorts him from the Emergency department comments that his ECG trace looks odd (Fig. 11.3):

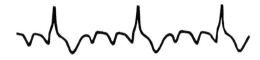

Fig. 11.3

(a) Can you tell him what the rhythm strip shows?
Atrial flutter with a 3 to 1 block.

(b) What will you suggest needs to be done?
This patient's cardiac failure has probably decompensated as a result of developing atrial fibrillation. Atrial flutter is generally resistant to drug treatment but easily reverts to sinus rhythm with a low energy (20 joule) DC cardioversion. This is indicated here.

11.4 You are asked to come urgently to see a 56-year-old man in the ward who is due to go to theatre for an appendicectomy. His rhythm appears to be irregular on the defibrillator monitor (Fig. 11.4). The anaesthetic registrar suggests that he has complete heart block and needs to be paced before going to theatre.

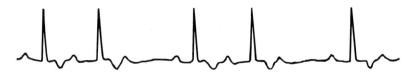

Fig. 11.4

(a) Do you agree with him?

No. The strip shows a Wenkebach second degree heart block (there is progressive prolongation of the PR interval with failure of conduction of every third atrial contraction).

(b) What will you suggest needs to be done?

This is usually a benign rhythm. It is generally due to high parasympathetic drive to the AV node. It is likely to respond to atropine and is unlikely to progress to complete heart block. No specific treatment is required; the patient can proceed urgently to theatre.

11.5 You are caring for a man after cardiac surgery who has epicardial pacing wires. You are told he is in AAI at 80 beats/minute.

What does AAI mean?

The atrium is paced, the atrium is sensed and the response to sensing is to inhibit pacing.

MINI-TUTORIAL

The chamber paced may be atrium (A), ventricle (V) or both/dual (D).
 The chamber sensed may be atrium (A), ventricle (V) or both/dual (D).
 The response to sensing may be inhibition of pacing (I), triggering of pacing (T) or both inhibition and triggering (D).
 In the latter case, sensing of a spontaneous atrial beat results in inhibition of atrial pacing but triggering of ventricular pacing (if no spontaneous beat occurs within a specified time).
 Commonly used modes are AAI, VVI and DDD.

11.6 The ECG strip in Fig. 11.5 is obtained in the Emergency department from a 67-year-old man with cardiomyopathy and a pacemaker. The registrar says that the patient had a DDD pacemaker.

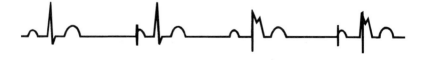

Fig. 11.5

(a) Do you agree?
Yes: both atrial and ventricular pacing spikes are observed. The first is a sinus beat which is normally conducted to the ventricle (both atrial and ventricular beat appropriately sensed and the pacemaker inhibited), and the second is an atrially paced beat which is normally conducted to the ventricle. The third is a spontaneous atrial beat which the pacemaker is sensing and is pacing the ventricle (in the absence of spontaneous ventricular activity within a specified period). The final beat is both atrially and ventricularly paced.

(b) Does the strip suggest that the pacemaker is working appropriately?
Yes. The pacemaker appears to be appropriately sensing and pacing.

11.7 You are urgently called to see a 75-year-old woman who has become bradycardic despite having a temporary transvenous ventricular pacing wire *in situ*. The rhythm strip of Fig. 11.6 has been run off for you.

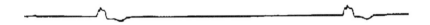

Fig. 11.6

(a) What do you think is happening?
There is a failure of the pacing spike to appear when expected. This is *failure to pace*.

(b) What will you do?
Quickly look at the pacing box. If the pacing box is functioning correctly then the pacing indicator should be regularly flashing. If there is no flashing then the battery may be dead or the box malfunctioning. If the sense indicator is regularly flashing rather than the pace indicator then this means that oversensing is the problem (the pacing box is picking up some electrical activity which it is inaccurately concluding is ventricular depolarisation). In this case, increasing the set value for the ventricular sensitivity may resolve the problem.

The commonest cause of failure to pace is a loose connection, or disconnection, of the pacing wire to the cable (which is easy to check rapidly). A faulty cable is unusual.

Unless the problem is very rapidly identifiable and correctable, in a patient with a rate as low as this it will be necessary to rapidly give isoprenaline to increase the rate or to institute cardiac massage and external pacing where the patient is unconscious.

11.8 A 52-year-old man is maintained on epicardial ventricular pacing following an aortic valve replacement. He is in atrial fibrillation and is paced in VVI mode. He has had an episode of syncope at which time the rhythm strip of Fig. 11.7 was recorded:

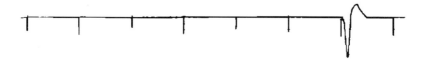

Fig. 11.7

(a) What do you think is the cause of his syncope?
Failure of the pacemaker to initiate a depolarisation or 'capture' the ventricle.

Failure to capture is recognised when there are clear pacing spikes without associated complexes indicating myocardial depolarisation.

(b) What will you do?
Possible manoeuvres to rectify the situation include increasing the output of the pacemaker or reversing the polarity of the pacing wires. However, the problem may be caused by failure of the wire to be in contact with the myocardium (more of a problem with recently placed transvenous wires) or the wire contacting with myocardium which is damaged and consequently not depolarisable. In these cases repositioning or replacing of wires may be required.

11.9 Every time an eldery woman coughs or moves her pacemaker is observed to stop pacing. A rhythm strip of such an event is available (Fig. 11.8):

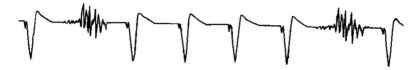

Fig. 11.8

What do you think is happening and what will you do to rectify the situation?
This is '*oversensing*'. The pacemaker is interpreting the interference as a beat. The sensitivity needs to be decreased (by setting the sensitivity to a higher figure). In this case there is obvious electrical activity on the trace, but sometimes the pacemaker may sense activity which is not well seen on the trace. Looking at the sense indicator on the pacing box should clarify the situation where the expected pacing is not occurring.

MINI-TUTORIAL

The *higher* the numerical value at which the sensitivity is set the *less* sensitive the pacemaker is to the patient's intrinsic electrical activity.
Appropriate initial (default) values for sensitivity are 0.5–0.6 mV for the atrium and 2.0–2.5 mV for the ventricle.

11.10 You are asked to look at the ECG strip from a patient with a VVI pacemaker because his pulse was noticed to be irregular (Fig. 11.9):

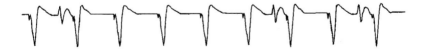

Fig. 11.9

What do you think is happening?
This is failure to sense. The pacemaker should be sensing the spontaneous ventricular beats and suppressing the subsequent pacemaker beat. Looking at the strip it is clear that the pacemaker rate continues regularly despite the occurrence of spontaneous beats.

The pacemaker should be adjusted to become more sensitive (a lower value for sensitivity should be set).

11.11 A patient on DDD pacing appears to be missing some ventricular paced beats, although atrial pacing appears consistent. You are asked if you think this might be due to 'crosstalk'.

Do you have any idea what crosstalk is? What will you say?
This can occur with A–V sequential pacemakers as a result of inappropriate sensing of the atrial output by the ventricular pacing circuit. The atrial activity is incorrectly interpreted as a QRS and ventricular output is inhibited. Consequently only atrial stimulation occurs without subsequent ventricular activation. The atrial pace and ventricular sense indicators will flash simultaneously. Crosstalk is more likely where the atrial and ventricular wires are placed close together, the atrial output is set high and the ventricular sensitivity is very sensitive (low number on the setting). If adjusting these does not correct the problem, then changing to VVI pacing avoids the problem.

11.12 You are asked to see a man who has gone into atrial fibrillation after cardiac surgery. He is in DDD pacing mode.

You are asked if you want to alter his pacing. What will you say?
Yes, this would be a good idea. Atrial capture is not possible in a patient in AF, making atrial pacing pointless; furthermore, there is risk of precipitating VT or VF if a patient is paced in DDD mode while in AF. This results from the fact that when a QRS arrives at the same time as an atrial pacing spike then that QRS cannot be sensed (this is intentional in the design of pacemakers to avoid crosstalk). Since the QRS is not sensed the subsequent ventricular pacing will occur 0.2 seconds after the unsensed QRS and will fall on the T wave, with the associated risk of provoking arrhythmia. Changing the pacing mode to VVI while the patient is in atrial fibrillation is appropriate.

12

Electrolyte interpretation

12.1 A 79-year-old woman is admitted to intensive care with a Glasgow Coma Score of 5. Her electrolyte result is phoned to the unit and is shown to you:

Sodium	158	(132–144 mmol/l
Potassium	4.9	(3.1–4.8 mmol/l)
Chloride	129	(93–108 mmol/l)
Bicarbonate	27	(21–32 mmol/l)
Glucose	61	(3.0–5.5 mmol/l)
Urea	24.0	(3.0–8.0 mmol/l)
Creatinine	160	(60–120 µmol/l)

(a) What observations do you make?
She has hyperglycaemic hyperosmolality.

Her glucose is markedly increased. The sodium is increased because the high glucose has caused an osmotic diuresis with relatively more water loss than saline.

MINI-TUTORIAL

Osmolality may be measured directly or can be calculated. Calculated osmolality is derived by doubling the sodium and adding the glucose and urea: $2 \times (Na) + glucose + urea$. In this case: $2 \times (158) + 61 + 24 = 401$.

Sometimes the measured osmolality (measured in the laboratory by depression of freezing point) will be higher than the calculated value due to the presence of extraneous substances with osmotic activity (e.g. mannitol, ethylene glycol, alcohol, methanol).

(b) What treatment will you suggest?
- Intravenous fluid – she is hyperosmolar, so she needs water, which is generally administered as 5% glucose.
- Low dose insulin infusion (1 IU/h) to slowly bring down the blood sugar, with frequent blood glucose monitoring and appropriate

dose adjustment. NOTE: minimal insulin rates are generally required in these hyperosmolar non-ketotic patients.

- Subcutaneous heparin – since she has an increased risk of thrombosis.
- General care for her in an unconscious state.

12.2 A 20-year-old man with a serious head injury has an increasing urine output. He has passed 790 ml over the last hour (and 490 ml the previous hour). His fluid intake has been restricted to 20 ml/h since admission. The following electrolyte results have just been reported:

Plasma

Sodium	162	(132–144 mmol/l)
Potassium	3.3	(3.1–4.8 mmol/l)
Chloride	128	(93–108 mmol/l)
Bicarbonate	27	(21–32 mmol/l)
Urea	10.0	(3.0–8.0 mmol/l)
Creatinine	120	(60–120 μmol/l)
Glucose	12.0	(3.0–5.5 mmol/l)
Osmolality	348	(280–295 mOsm/l) (measured)

Urine

Sodium	< 5	(mmol/l)
Osmolality	128	(mOsm/l) (measured)

(a) You are asked why you think he is putting out so much urine.
This man has high serum osmolality (i.e. too little serum water) and should therefore be producing small amounts of hyperosmolar (concentrated) urine. He is not. The hormone which controls urine concentration is ADH (high ADH = small volume concentrated urine, low ADH = high volume dilute urine). In this case there is inadequate ADH and the diagnosis is diabetes insipidus. In ICU diabetes insipidus (DI) is usually seen in the setting of brain death.

(NOTE: Diabetes mellitus causes both plasma and urine osmolality to be *high* due to the high glucose content.)

(b) Formal testing confirms brain death and diabetes insipidus. His relatives have consented to organ donation, but the surgical team will not arrive for another eight hours. He has passed 690 ml of colourless urine in the last hour. You are asked what you want to do. What will you suggest?

You may wish to confirm that the urine is of low osmolality in the face of increased plasma osmolality (so checking of urine and plasma osmolality is appropriate). In any polyuric patient you should exclude significant glycosuria (which is likely in this situation if the patient has been severely stressed during the process of brain death and has been given intravenous glucose).

The finding of a high plasma osmolality with low urinary osmolality confirms the diagnosis of diabetes insipidus.

Diabetes insipidus is treated by replacement of ADH with synthetic ADH (d-desamino arginine vasopressin: DDAVP). Small doses intravenously have a rapid effect (0.2 μg is a reasonable starting dose).

MINI-TUTORIAL

Giving 5% glucose rapidly to correct the hypernatraemia (without ddAVP) in patients with diabetes insipidus invariably leads to hyperglycaemia and glycosuria, which results in an unhelpful osmotic diuresis and further dehydration.

It is important to diagnose DI early before patients dehydrate themselves. Urine outputs of > 200 ml/h should make you suspicious in severely brain injured patients.

12.3 An 85-year-old man has been bedridden for three days in assisted accommodation with a pneumonia. The following electrolyte results are obtained:

Plasma

Sodium	171	(132–144 mmol/l)
Potassium	3.8	(3.1–4.8 mmol/l)
Chloride	134	(93–108 mmol/l)
Bicarbonate	37	(21–32 mmol/l)
Urea	35	(3.0–8.0 mmol/l)
Creatinine	200	(60–120 μmol/l)
Glucose	5.0	(3.0–5.5 mmol/l)

Urine

Sodium	< 5	(mmol/l)
Osmolality	924	(mOsm/l) (measured)

The medical registrar says that he thinks the man is 'dry', hasn't taken much fluid orally and has had inadequate intravenous fluid. He says that the urine is consistent with this diagnosis.

Do you agree?
Yes. The patient is hyperosmolar. Calculated osmolality = (2 × Na + urea + glucose) = 342 + 35 + 5 = 382). The urine sodium is low due to increased sodium reabsorption in response to low intravascular volume, so the very high urinary osmolality is appropriate as the patient is maximally attempting to retain water in the face of his plasma hyperosmolality.

12.4 A sixty-year-old lady suffers a convulsion (in another hospital) four days after having a laparotomy for a radical hysterectomy. She suffered hypotension during her operation and has received 2000 ml 5% glucose daily since her operation. Following intubation her fitting is controlled by diazepam. She is transferred to your ICU.
    Her electrolytes are as follows:

Plasma

Sodium	109	(132–144 mmol/l)
Potassium	1.7	(3.1–4.8 mmol/l)
Chloride	77	(93–108 mmol/l)
Bicarbonate	25	(21–32 mmol/l)
Glucose	5.1	(3.0–5.5 mmol/l)
Urea	2.9	(3.0–8.0 mmol/l)
Creatinine	60	(60–120 μmol/l)
Osmolality	226	(280–295 mOsm/l)

Urine

Sodium	43	(mmol/l)
Osmolality	253	(mOsm/l)

The surgeon says he has no idea why she has had a fit and thinks she must have had a cerebro-vascular accident (CVA).

Is any alternative cause suggested by the electrolytes?
Yes. The electrolytes show hyponatraemia and hypo-osmolality consistent with water intoxication. Water is not being excreted by the kidney (the urine osmolality is higher than the plasma), which is not appropriate in the face of low osmolality (the urine osmolality should be lower than plasma osmolality when water is being excreted).

MINI-TUTORIAL

Following surgical stress ADH secretion is increased (e.g. pain, when opiates increase secretion) and water loads are excreted poorly, especially by women. Consequently water loads (as represented by 5% glucose) should be avoided or used with care.

Hyponatraemia with hypo-osmolality is very dangerous. Patients with hyponatraemia are at risk of convulsions and respiratory arrest; subsequently they are likely to suffer severe neurological handicap.

Arieff (1991) described the picture:

- 15 women, mean age 41, pre-operative sodium 138 mmol/l.
- An average of 49 h later the mean sodium of the group was 108 mmol/l.
- The urine sodium and osmolality were high – mean sodium 68 mmol/l, osmolality 501 mOsm/l.
- Grand mal seizures and respiratory arrest occurred.
- The subsequent rate of correction of the sodium was < 0.7 mmol/l/h.
- Seven patients recovered from coma but relapsed 2–6 days later.
- 27% died, 13% had limb paralysis and 60% persistent vegetative state.

The neurological damage is associated with central nervous system demyelination. While the relationship between treatment and neurological deterioration is unclear it is recommended that sodium levels are not increased at greater than 2 mmol/l/h and that sodium levels are not permitted to overshoot (i.e. to become > 135 mmol/l).

Arieff A. Hyponatraemia, convulsions, respiratory arrest and permanent brain damage after elective surgery in healthy women. *N. Engl. J. Med.* 1986; **314**: 24.
Arieff A. Treatment of symptomatic hyponatremia: Neither haste nor waste. *Crit. Care Med.* 1991; **19**: 748–51.

12.5 A 73-year-old lady is admitted with confusion. She is hypotensive and is clinically dehydrated with poor skin turgor. She has been taking chlorthiazide and digoxin. In the emer-

gency department she is noted to have severe hyponatraemia and her urine and serum osmolalities are measured.
Her electrolytes are as follows:

Plasma

Sodium	110	(132–144 mmol/l)
Potassium	3.0	(3.1–4.8 mmol/l)
Chloride	80	(93–108 mmol/l)
Bicarbonate	19	(21–32 mmol/l)
Glucose	8.2	(3.0–5.5 mmol/l)
Urea	16	(3.0–8.0 mmol/l)
Creatinine	140	(60–120 μmol/l)
Osmolality	242	(280–295 mOsm/l)

Urine

Sodium	72	(mmol/l)
Osmolality	502	(mOsm/l)

The Emergency registrar thinks the patient has SIADH. Do you agree?
No. This lady has biochemical features of syndrome of inappropriate anti-diuretic hormone (SIADH), *but* the diagnosis cannot be made in the face of volume depletion or diuretic treatment.

This lady has low serum osmolality and should be excreting a dilute urine to get rid of the excess water. She is clearly not doing this, since her urine is very concentrated (high sodium > 20 mmol/l and high osmolality).

To make a confident diagnosis of syndrome of inappropriate anti-diuretic hormone (SIADH) it is necessary to rule out clinical fluid depletion and diuretic therapy. Most patients presenting with this electrolyte picture are elderly, are on diuretics and are clinically hypovolaemic (the ADH response is an *appropriate* response to their intravascular volume deficiency).

Stopping the diuretic and cautious administration of normal saline (so as not to raise the sodium and osmolality too rapidly or to provoke left ventricular failure) generally resolves the situation.

12.6 An insulin dependent diabetic with renal failure on chronic dialysis is admitted to ICU in a semi-conscious state. Her electrolyte results are as follows:

Sodium	95	(132–144 mmol/l)
Potassium	6.5	(3.1–4.8 mmol/l)
Chloride	68	(93–108 mmol/l)
Bicarbonate	15	(21–32 mmol/l)
Glucose	110	(3.0–5.5 mmol/l)
Urea	28.0	(3.0–8.0 mmol/l)
Creatinine	370	(60–120 µmol/l)
Osmolality	333	(280–295 mOsm/l) (measured)

There has been a bit of a dispute in the Emergency department. The registrar thought that since her osmolality was so high she should be given half normal saline, while the medical registrar felt that twice normal saline was indicated in view of her low sodium. Both are up when she arrives in ICU!

(a) How will you treat the hyponatraemia?
This girl has hyper-osmolar hypernatraemia due to her very high glucose. The treatment for her hyponatraemia is insulin, which will also correct her hyperosmolality.

MINI-TUTORIAL

Hyponatraemia can be classified into several types:

- *Artefact*
  Sampling from a vein into which a 5% glucose infusion is running.
- *Pseudohyponatraemia*
  Abnormally high lipids or protein reducing water content of plasma (only affects 'indirectly' reading machines, these are the larger – main laboratory – machines, sodiums on blood gas machines read correctly in the presence of protein or lipid).
- *Hypo-osmolar hyponatraemia*
  The usual sort with low osmolality.
- *Hyper-osmolar hyponatraemia*
  Low sodium due to intra-cellular to extra-cellular fluid shifts caused by the high osmotic gradient pulling water out of cells.

In hyper-osmolar hyponatraemia a rough estimate of the 'true' sodium can be calculated by dividing the glucose by 3 and adding this to the measured sodium. In the case above this gives a corrected sodium result of 135, which is within normal limits.

There are other more complex formulae, such as:

$$\frac{sodium + glucose - 5.6}{5.6} \times 1.6$$

However, the more complex formulae do not lend themselves to quick mental calculation at bedside, and add little to the usefulness of the estimate in the clinical context.

12.7 You are treating a newly diagnosed 10-year-old with diabetic ketoacidosis. He has been given normal saline with potassium and an insulin infusion (4 u/h). It is noted that his sodium has risen to 152 mmol/l. A registrar from the Emergency department suggests that you should not have let this happen and suggests that it is because you have given the child normal saline.

	2 p.m.	4 p.m.	6 p.m.	
Sodium	144	150	152	(132–144 mmol/l)
Potassium	4.8	4.5	3.9	(3.1–4.8 mmol/l)
Chloride	108	116	122	(93–108 mmol/l)
Bicarbonate	5	5	8	(21–32 mmol/l)
Glucose	26	12	10	(3.0–5.5 mmol/l)
Urea	9.2	8.1	9.0	(3.0–8.0 mmol/l)
Creatinine	125	118	117	(60–120 μmol/l)
Osmolality (calc.)	323	320	323	(280–295 mOsm/l)
Anion gap	34	33.5	26	
Adjusted sodium (approx.)	153	154	155	

Do you agree?

No. Because of the high extra-cellular glucose the first sodium result is reduced as a consequence of osmotic movement from the cells to the extra-cellular space. When the sodium is adjusted the sodium is 153 mmol/l, at which level it remains on subsequent measurements (approximately).

The second question relates to whether maintaining the sodium at this level is a bad thing. The osmolality is the important measurement. In this case the osmolality remains unchanged (since the sodium rises as the glucose falls). It is probably undesirable for the osmolality to be altered rapidly, and this effect on the sodium is probably useful to prevent rapid changes as glucose levels fall.

MINI-TUTORIAL

Cerebral oedema is a well recognised, and feared, complication of diabetic ketoacidosis in children, often resulting in death.

While the exact cause remains unclear, it is recommended that sodium levels should rise during rehydration. Falling sodium levels may be a marker of excessive free water administration.

Mel JM, Werther GA. Incidence and outcome of diabetic cerebral oedema in childhood: Are there predictors? *Paediatr. Child Health* 1995; **31**: 17–20.

12.8 You are reviewing a woman of 54 with severe chronic liver disease. She has ascites and peripheral muscle wasting. Having examined the patient and biochemistry results the intensive care specialist suggests that her renal function may not be so good. On checking her creatinine clearance this proves to be the case.

Sodium	136	(132–144 mmol/l)
Potassium	4.4	(3.1–4.8 mmol/l)
Chloride	107	(93–108 mmol/l)
Bicarbonate	22	(21–32 mmol/l)
Urea	14.8	(3.0–8.0 mmol/l)
Creatinine	130	(60–120 μmol/l)
Creatinine clearance	0.32	(1.5–2.5 ml/s)

What is it about her condition and her biochemistry which suggests that her renal function is poor?
A patient with severe hepatic dysfunction would be expected to have a low urea (impaired hepatic synthesis) and someone with low muscle bulk has a low production rate for creatinine which should result in a low plasma level in the face of normal renal function. The high normal levels of urea and creatinine in this clinical situation are highly suggestive of poor renal function; indeed, normal levels may

be associated with significant impairment of renal function in patients with significant hepatic disease. The creatinine clearance will appropriately reflect renal function in the face of either or both hepatic disease and low muscle bulk.

12.9 You are asked to review a patient on the surgical ward who has become hypotensive. It looks like he has been septic for a few days. He has been 'nil by mouth' for four days but has had 2000 ml intravenously each day. The man has a dry tongue but appears to have an elevated JVP.

Urea	22.6	(3.0–8.0 mmol/l)
Creatinine	120	(60–120 μmol/l)

While you are discussing the fluid status with the ICU specialist he asks you if the urea:creatinine ratio is consistent with intravascular fluid depletion.

Is it?
Yes. The ratio is high, suggesting volume depletion.

MINI-TUTORIAL

Volume depletion and a protein load in the bowel (usually blood) are the two causes of a discrepancy between the urea and creatinine where the urea is higher than would be expected from the creatinine. In this case the creatinine is at the upper range of normality, while the urea is more than twice normal.

12.10 A man is admitted unconscious to ICU from the Emergency department. He is unkempt and the Emergency registrar has considered head injury. He has had a CT of his head, which is completely normal. A number of pathology tests have been done while he was in the Emergency department and the results accompany him to the ward:

Plasma

Sodium	143	(132–144 mmol/l)
Potassium	4.0	(3.1–4.8 mmol/l)
Chloride	105	(93–108 mmol/l)

Bicarbonate	17	(21–32 mmol/l)
Glucose	5.0	(3.0–5.5 mmol/l)
Urea	3.6	(3.0–8.0 mmol/l)
Creatinine	60	(60–120 μmol/l)
Osmolality	375	(280–295 mOsm/l)

Urine   negative for ketones

(a) The medical registrar says the patient has a massive anion gap. Do you know what he is talking about? Do you agree with him?
Yes. This patient has a large anion gap of 30.

MINI-TUTORIAL

Anion gap = 'unmeasured anions'

Anion gap = $(Na^+ + K^+) - (Cl^- + HCO_3^-)$

Metabolic acidosis (reduction of bicarbonate) must be associated with either an increase of the anion gap (anion gap acidosis) or of the chloride (non-anion gap or hyperchloraemic acidosis), since the overall quantity of cations and anions must match (see Fig. 12.1).

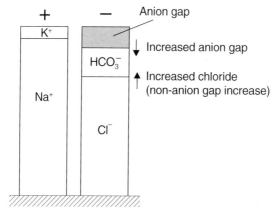

Fig. 12.1

Bicarbonate loss from the gut or kidney with replacement by chloride containing fluid will result in a non-anion gap or hyperchloraemic acidosis.

Conditions for which anions may be increased to cause an increased anion gap include:

- lactic acidosis
- ketoacidosis
- renal failure (only when severe = creatinine > 400 µmol/l)
- toxin ingestion – inc. salicylate, ethylene glycol, methanol, pyro-glutamic acid.

(b) The medical registrar also says he thinks the patient has taken an overdose, since the osmolality is 375 mOsm/l. What is he talking about now? Do you agree with him this time?

The calculated osmolality is normal (295 mOsm/l), so the high measured osmolality (375 mOsm/l) is not due to sodium, glucose or urea.

There is an osmolar gap (calculated osmolality minus measured osmolality) of 80.

Things that cause an osmolar gap include ethanol, methanol, ethylene glycol (anti-freeze) and mannitol.

12.11 A young woman is admitted to the Emergency department. She is hyperventilating. A medical student says he can smell ketones on her breath. Her electrolytes are as follows:

Plasma

Sodium	137	(132–144 mmol/l)	
Potassium	4.0	(3.1–4.8 mmol/l)	
Chloride	105	(93–108 mmol/l)	
Bicarbonate	29	(21–32 mmol/l)	
pH	7.60	(7.35–7.42)	
P_aCO_2	28	(35–45 mmHg)	3.72 kPa
P_aO_2	128	(80–100 mmHg)	17.02 kPa

Are the arterial blood gases consistent with a diagnosis of diabetic ketoacidosis?

The pH reveals an alkalosis. There is no anion gap to suggest a metabolic acidosis (e.g. lactic acid or ketoacidosis). The alkalosis is due to respiratory alkalosis/hyperventilation (the P_aCO_2 is low).

The student must be imagining the ketones.

12.12 A 23-year-old man has been treated for diabetic ketoacidosis. On the day after admission he is noted to be still hyperventilating and his electrolytes show that the bicarbonate is still low. The medical registrar states that the ketoacidosis is not resolved and that intravenous insulin will need to continue. He also suggests that you have inadequately treated him.

	Admission	36 h later	
Sodium	137	139	(132–144 mmol/l)
Potassium	6.1	4.9	(3.1–4.8 mmol/l)
Chloride	94	117	(93–108 mmol/l)
Bicarbonate	7	15	(21–32 mmol/l)
Glucose	39	5.2	(3.0–5.5 mmol/l)
Urea	18.1	11.1	(3.0–8.0 mmol/l)
Creatinine	219	146	(60–120 μmol/l)

Is the registrar correct?
No.

On admission the anion gap is 42. The large anion gap is to be expected in a case of severe ketoacidosis. The ketones would be expected to be present in large quantity in both the urine and the blood.

Following treatment the anion gap is 12. This is within normal limits. The metabolic picture is now a hyperchloraemic non-anion gap metabolic acidosis. This has probably resulted from a generous use of intravenous sodium chloride for resuscitation. It is of little significance and is likely to be rectified by the patient within a few hours. In the absence of a raised anion gap there are unlikely to be significant residual ketones and urine testing will confirm this. Continuing the insulin infusion with the aim of treating the acidosis is not appropriate.

There is no evidence that the treatment of the patient's ketoacidosis has been inadequate.

12.13 A 52-year-old woman is admitted to the Emergency department. She is hyperventilating. The registrar from the Emergency department suggests that she has respiratory alkalosis with a compensating metabolic acidosis. Her electrolytes are as follows:

Plasma

Sodium	125	(132–144 mmol/l)	
Potassium	5.2	(3.1–4.8 mmol/l)	
Chloride	86	(93–108 mmol/l)	
Bicarbonate	20	(21–32 mmol/l)	
pH	7.64	(7.35–7.42)	
P_aCO_2	16.7	(35–45 mmHg)	2.22 kPa
P_aO_2	104	(80–100 mmHg)	13.83 kPa

Do you agree?

No. There is certainly respiratory alkalosis and the anion gap is raised (24); however, metabolic compensation is not associated with an increased anion gap (this is caused by one of the causes of increased anion already discussed). In this case the bicarbonate is 20, but would be 29 if the reduction associated with the increased anion gap is taken into account; there is therefore no metabolic compensation for the respiratory alkalosis. (This woman turned out to have ketoacidosis, but with a profound anxiety state which resulted in her hyperventilation in response to her illness.)

12.14 A 20-year-old woman is brought to the Emergency department having been found unconscious at home. The emergency registrar says that she thinks this woman has taken a salicylate overdose. Her electrolyte and blood gas results are as follows:

Sodium	135	(132–144 mmol/l)	
Potassium	2.6	(3.1–4.8 mmol/l)	
Chloride	94	(93–108 mmol/l)	
Bicarbonate	14	(21–32 mmol/l)	
Glucose	12.2	(3.0–5.5 mmol/l)	
Urea	12.5	(3.0–8.0 mmol/l)	
Creatinine	180	(60–120 μmol/l)	
Osmolality	295	(280–295 mOsm/l)	
pH	7.48	(7.35–7.42)	
P_aCO_2	19	(35–45 mmHg)	2.53 kPa
P_aO_2	102	(80–100 mmHg)	13.57 kPa

Is there biochemical support for the diagnosis of salicylate toxicity?

Yes. This girl has a large anion gap, so she has a metabolic acidosis consistent with salicylate ingestion. Salicylate has a direct stimulatory effect on the respiratory centre, so the hyperventilation (respiratory alkalosis) is greater than would be predicted as a compensation for the metabolic acidosis and results in a net alkalosis. These results are thus entirely consistent with salicylate toxicity; salicylate levels need to be measured.

12.15 A man is referred to intensive care because he is increasingly confused and his urine output has reduced. The ICU registrar tells you that this is a really interesting case because there are both acidosis and alkalosis at the same time. The electrolytes are as follows:

Plasma

Sodium	138	(132–144 mmol/l)
Potassium	2.7	(3.1–4.8 mmol/l)
Chloride	71	(93–108 mmol/l)
Bicarbonate	45	(21–32 mmol/l)

Do you agree with her?

Yes, this is an example of metabolic acidosis co-existing with metabolic alkalosis. It is actually quite common.

The high bicarbonate indicates a *metabolic alkalosis*. Metabolic alkalosis is common in sick patients due to potassium depletion (hydrogen ions enter cells to maintain electrical neutrality when K^+ is not available; HCO_3^- remains extra-cellularly) and volume depletion (HCO_3^- is reabsorbed from the tubular fluid when sodium is maximally reabsorbed, since there is inadequate chloride to be reabsorbed with all of the sodium). There is an increased anion gap (of 25) which indicates a *metabolic acidosis*.

MINI-TUTORIAL

When metabolic alkalosis and metabolic acidosis co-exist the pH may be normal, even though the acid base status is grossly upset.

12.16 A hypotensive woman with an intra-abdominal abscess is admitted to ICU with the following electrolyte and blood gas results:

Sodium	121	(132–144 mmol/l)	
Potassium	3.0	(3.1–4.8 mmol/l)	
Chloride	68	(93–108 mmol/l)	
Bicarbonate	33	(21–32 mmol/l)	
Glucose	5.3	(3.0–5.5 mmol/l)	
Urea	15.7	(3.0–8.0 mmol/l)	
Creatinine	90	(60–120 μmol/l)	
pH	7.68	(7.35–7.42)	
P_aCO_2	37	(35–45 mmHg)	4.92 kPa
P_aO_2	179	(80–100 mmHg)	23.81 kPa

The medical registrar says that her electrolyte results show a triple acid base disturbance. What is he on about now? Do you agree with him?
This lady is alkalotic, as can be seen by looking at her pH and this is metabolic, as her P_aCO_2 is within normal range. She has an increased anion gap (23) so by definition has a metabolic acidosis (note how a pre-existing metabolic alkalosis can mask this if you just look at the blood gas results and not the electrolytes – in this lady marked vomiting has caused her alkalosis). She has a pH of 7.68 and so should be under-ventilating to compensate. She is not hypo-ventilating, so has an inappropriate respiratory alkalosis. This is termed a triple acid base disturbance.

12.17 A man with severe congestive cardiac failure and COAD (FEV$_1$ 500 ml) is admitted to ICU with an acute exacerbation of his respiratory disease. The following electrolyte and blood gas results are obtained:

Sodium	136	(132–144 mmol/l)
Potassium	4.0	(3.1–4.8 mmol/l)
Chloride	85	(93–108 mmol/l)
Bicarbonate	24	(21–32 mmol/l)
Glucose	6.3	(3.0–5.5 mmol/l)
Urea	12.7	(3.0–8.0 mmol/l)

Creatinine	220	(60–120 μmol/l)	
pH	7.20	(7.35–7.42)	
P_aCO_2	62	(35–45 mmHg)	8.25 kPa
P_aO_2	64	(80–100 mmHg)	8.51 kPa

The medical registrar is a bit confused because this man has been recorded as being a CO_2 retainer on past admissions, but this time the bicarbonate is normal.

Can you help her?
The bicarbonate has been reduced as a consequence of a metabolic acidosis (evidenced by an increased anion gap).

This man is acidotic, as can be seen by looking at his pH, and this is both metabolic (increased anion gap = 31) and respiratory, as his P_aCO_2 is above the normal range. The bicarbonate is not as low as would be expected from the degree of the anion gap. The gap is increased by 19 (31 minus the normal gap of about 12) and the bicarbonate level is usually reduced by the same amount as the anion gap is increased. So if his bicarbonate started at 30 then we would expect a level of 11 (30 – 19) with this degree of acidosis. In this case the bicarbonate before the acidosis developed must have been 24 + 19 = 43, a marked metabolic alkalosis as a consequence of compensation for CO_2 retention.

12.18 A 16-year-old boy was admitted with ketoacidosis. On arrival he had poor skin turgor and a dry tongue but was not hypotensive (120/80). In the Emergency department he received 1 litre of normal saline over 30 minutes and was catheterised. On catheterisation there was 500 ml urine in the bladder and he has passed 30 ml of urine subsequently.

He is rapidly transferred to ICU since several cases are expected in EMD from a road accident.

His electrolyte and blood gas results are as follows:

Sodium	123	(132–144 mmol/l)
Potassium	5.6	(3.1–4.8 mmol/l)
Chloride	80	(93–108 mmol/l)
Bicarbonate	4	(21–32 mmol/l)
Glucose	25.3	(3.0–5.5 mmol/l)
Urea	14.7	(3.0–8.0 mmol/l)

| Creatinine | 207 | (60–120 μmol/l) |
| Osmolality | 290 | (280–295 mOsm/l) |

(a) As he arrives you note that the normal saline is almost through. What treatments will you give to him?
Intravenous insulin has been shown to result in better control in diabetic ketoacidosis (DKA) than does intra-muscular insulin (particularly when patients are shocked). Subcutaneous insulin is contraindicated in shocked patients, as uptake is very erratic. Normal saline is used as the initial resuscitation fluid and potassium supplements are indicated, even when initial levels show hyperkalaemia, as total body potassium is low and plasma levels drop rapidly as soon as the insulin is started. In general terms, if patients with DKA have a urine output then potassium supplementation should be considered. Sodium bicarbonate is rarely, if ever, indicated.

MINI-TUTORIAL

Patients with diabetic ketoacidosis (DKA) who receive $NaHCO_3$ show delay in the improvement of ketosis when compared with controls. Alkali administration augments ketone production and does not appear to be beneficial in DKA. Hypokalaemia is liable to be exacerbated by bicarbonate administration.

Green SM, Rothrock SG, Ho JD, Gallant RD, Borger R, Thomas TL, Zimmerman G. Failure of adjunctive bicarbonate to improve outcome in severe pediatric diabetic ketoacidosis. *J. Ann. Emerg. Med.* 1998; **31**(1): 41–8.
Okuda Y, Adrogue HJ, Field JB, Nohara H, Yamashita K. Counterproductive effects of sodium bicarbonate in diabetic ketoacidosis. *J. Clin. Endocrinol. Metab.* 1996; **81**(1): 314–20.

At 6 p.m. the patient's blood sugar is noted to be 10 mmol/l. It is suggested to you that the insulin should be switched off.

(b) What do you think?
No. This error results from a fixation that the fundamental role of the insulin infusion is to treat the hyperglycaemia rather than to address the ketoacidosis. The insulin infusion should be continued until the ketoacidosis has resolved. A glucose infusion will usually be required to avoid hypoglycaemia during the latter stages of the infusion.

When the insulin infusion is stopped too early the ketoacidosis rapidly recurs.

12.19 A patient with a high output small bowel fistula is referred to ICU due to increasing tachypnoea. His electrolytes and blood gas results show:

Sodium	132	(132–144 mmol/l)
Potassium	3.0	(3.1–4.8 mmol/l)
Chloride	110	(93–108 mmol/l)
Bicarbonate	15	(21–32 mmol/l)
Urea	20.2	(3.0–8.0 mmol/l)
Creatinine	140	(60–120 μmol/l)
pH	7.26	(7.35–7.42)
$P_a CO_2$	32	(35–45 mmHg) 4.26 kPa

What is the likely cause of this metabolic picture?
There is an acidosis (pH = 7.26) but no anion gap: $(Na^+ + K^+) - (Cl^- + HCO_3^-)$ $(132 + 3) - (110 + 15) = 10$. This is hyperchloraemic non-anion gap metabolic acidosis. The likely cause is loss of bicarbonate rich fluid from his small bowel fistula. He needs fluid replacement with potassium, and bicarbonate is also appropriate since this has been lost. The prognosis in hyperchloraemic non-anion gap metabolic acidosis is much better than where there is an anion gap due to lactic acidosis.

12.20 You are rung urgently when the following results are phoned from the laboratory at 7 a.m. The patient has rapid AF and has been moved to coronary care for cardioversion. The electrolytes were being checked prior to the cardioversion. His previous potassium result was 3.5, but that was 3 months ago. He has been on a thiazide diuretic. The night intern asks your advice about how rapidly intravenous potassium can be administered.

Sodium	136	(132–144 mmol/l)
Potassium	1.6	(3.1–4.8 mmol/l)
Chloride	108	(93–108 mmol/l)
Bicarbonate	31	(21–32 mmol/l)

What will you tell her?
The blood results cannot be correct.

The anion gap is negative (−1.4). Negative anion gaps are not possible, so the results must be wrong. Either a laboratory error (likely at 7 a.m. in the morning at change-over) or a transcription error has occurred. In this case it was a simple case of misreading a potassium of 4.6 as 1.6 on the telephoned result.

12.21 While you are assisting with the care of a sick man on the surgical ward some arterial blood gas results arrive. The results show that he has a pH of 7.2 and a bicarbonate of 13 mmol/l. The lactate is 6.7 mmol/l. The surgical registrar states that 'he needs some bicarbonate'. A medical student who observes this asks you 'When should you give bicarbonate?' and 'How does it help?'.

What will you tell her?
In patients with metabolic acidosis due to lactic acidosis (the usual cause in sick, hypotensive, hypoxic patients) there is no evidence that the administration of bicarbonate is beneficial, and it may be detrimental. Treatment aimed at the underlying cause (sepsis, low cardiac output, etc.) is much more appropriate.

Sodium bicarbonate is useful in the acute management of severe hyperkalaemia and tricyclic overdose. It is used in the generation of an alkaline diuresis in salicylate overdose and rhabdomyolysis.

MINI-TUTORIAL

Lactic acidosis decreases left ventricular contractility, but bicarbonate infusion does not directly increase left ventricular contractility during lactic acidaemia. Nor does bicarbonate improve haemodynamic variables in patients with lactic acidosis.

Cooper DJ, Herbertson MJ, Werner HA, Walley KR. Bicarbonate does not increase left ventricular contractility during L-lactic acidemia in pigs. *Am. Rev. Respir. Dis.* 1993; **148**(2): 317–22.

Mathieu D, Neviere R, Billard V, Fleyfel M, Wattel F. Effects of bicarbonate therapy on hemodynamics and tissue oxygenation in patients with lactic acidosis: a prospective, controlled clinical study. *Crit. Care Med.* 1991; **19**(11): 1352–6.

12.22 A patient with known non-insulin-dependent diabetes is admitted to ICU with an infective exacerbation of COAD. He is ventilated and is treated with antibiotics, bronchodilators and

hydrocortisone with good effect. A routine blood sugar level (BSL) is 13.5 mmol/l.

Do you want to treat it?

Yes. There is good evidence that blood sugar levels in excess of 12.5 are associated with increased rates of infection and metabolic disturbance.

An insulin infusion is generally the favoured method of blood sugar control in ICU. In a previously non-insulin-dependent patient an initial rate of 1 unit per hour would be a reasonable starting point.

MINI-TUTORIAL

Maintaining blood glucose levels below 11 mmol/l following open heart surgery resulted in a decrease in the proportion of patients with deep wound infections, from 2.4% (24/990) to 1.5% (9/595) ($P < 0.02$) (Zerr et al., 1997).

Surgical patients who have one or more episodes of hyperglycaemia (> 12.1 mmol/l) on the first post-operative day experienced 5.7 times the 'serious' post-operative infection rate (excluding minor infections such as UTI) as did those who do not have hyperglycaemia during this period (Pomposelli et al., 1998).

Pomposelli JJ, Baxter JK, Babineau TJ, Pomfret EA, Driscoll DF, Forse RA, Bistrian BR. Early postoperative glucose control predicts nosocomial infection rate in diabetic patients. *J. Parenter. Enteral. Nutr.* 1998; **22**(2): 77–81.

Zerr KJ, Furnary AP, Grunkemeier GL, Bookin S, Kanhere V, Starr A. Glucose control lowers the risk of wound infection in diabetics after open heart operations. *Ann. Thorac. Surg.* 1997; **63**(2): 356–61.

12.23 A 70-year-old lady who has been slow to recover from pneumonia has her thyroid function tested. When tested she is still ventilated and has significant bi-basal consolidation. Her results are as follows:

T3 free	1.7	pmol/l	(2.4–5.4 pmol/l)
T4 free	6.2	pmol/l	(9–26 pmol/l
TSH	21	mU/l	(0.3–5 mU/l)

There is some discussion about these results, and it is suggested that they represent a 'sick euthyroid' picture.

(a) Do you agree?

No. The low T3 and T4 are consistent with sick euthyroid syndrome, but the TSH should also be low or normal. Here the TSH is very high, suggesting hypothyroidism.

(b) What treatment is indicated?

In patients with the sick euthryoid thyroid function picture (low T3, low T4, low or normal TSH) there is currently no evidence that treatment with thyroid hormone is of benefit.

In cases of hypothyroidism (indicated by high TSH values) thyroid hormone replacement is indicated. Since conversion of T4 to T3 is poor in sick patients, administration of T3 may be appropriate.

MINI-TUTORIAL

The commonest 'sick euthyroid' picture is one of low T3, but with normal TSH, total and free T4 levels. The low T3 levels are thought to be due to reduced conversion of T4 to T3. There is increased conversion to meta-bolically inactive reverse T3 (rT3). In sicker patients both T3 and T4 levels are usually reduced, while TSH levels are normal or low.

A high TSH is very unusual in critically ill patients and indicates primary hypothyroidism. Medications used in ICU frequently suppress TSH responses (particularly dopamine and glucocorticoids) and may complicate the diagnosis of hypothyroidism.

Camacho PM, Dwarkanathan AA. Sick euthyroid syndrome – What to do when thyroid function tests are abnormal in critically ill patients. *Postgraduate Med.* 1999; **105**(4): 215–19.

13

Haematology

13.1 You admit a man of 54 to intensive care following coronary artery grafting. He has significant ongoing post-operative bleeding (70–90 ml/h). Haematology results are as follows:

INR	2.6
APTT	60 sec
Hb	82 g/l
Platelets	$49 \times 10^9/l$

As the results arrive the surgeon phones and enquires if there is any medical reason for the bleeding.

What will you say?
There certainly is.

The prothrombin time (INR) is prolonged and requires Fresh Frozen Plasma (FFP) to correct it.

The APTT is prolonged, most likely due to residual heparin effect. This can be checked and/or additional protamine can be administered.

The platelet count is low and this may contribute to inadequate haemostasis. Platelet transfusion may reduce the rate of haemorrhage.

13.2 A 75-year-old man with known chronic liver disease is admitted from the Emergency department with a massive haematemesis. He has had an urgent gastroscopy and has been found to have a large pre-pyloric ulcer but no varices. His INR is 5.6, for which he has been given vitamin K (10 mg iv). His haemoglobin is 72 g/l and a blood transfusion is in progress.

(a) What further medical treatment will you feel is indicated?
Vitamin K is likely to improve the INR towards 1 (although it will usually remain somewhat abnormal in a patient with significant liver disease). However, this will take a few days. In the face of acute

bleeding the grossly abnormal INR (> 5) needs to be rapidly rectified. Infusion of Fresh Frozen Plasma (usually about 4 units) will be required to do this.

A patient with chronic liver disease with a major bleed is at risk of encephalopathy (especially if there is a prior history of encephalopathy). Lactulose (± neomycin) is indicated to reduce the risk of encephalopathy.

13.3 You are managing a 72-year-old man who has a pneumonia complicating his chronic renal failure. He has been 'haemofiltered', but this has been ceased while a tracheostomy is performed. There is significant ongoing bleeding from the tracheostomy site. Tests of coagulation (APTT and PT) are normal and he has a platelet count of 110 × 10⁹/l. The ICU consultant suggests giving DDAVP.

What is the rationale behind this request?
D-desamino arginine vasopressin (DDAVP) is a synthetic derivative of antidiuretic hormone. In addition to antidiuretic effect it has been shown to exert effects on bleeding including increases of plasma levels of factor VIII and von Willebrand factor (vWF).

MINI-TUTORIAL

Patients with uraemia commonly have a prolonged bleeding time which can be reversed by DDAVP.

DDAVP has been shown to reduce bleeding effectively in patients with mild haemophilia A or von Willebrand's disease. Initial observations that blood loss after cardiac surgery was markedly reduced by DDAVP have not been confirmed in later studies (which still indicate a blood loss reduction, but which is not clinically significant).

Mannucci PM. Desmopressin (DDAVP) in the treatment of bleeding disorders: the first 20 years. *Blood* 1997: **90**: 2515–21.

13.4 A consultant anaesthetist speaks to you about a patient in ICU whom he anaesthetised. The patient has had a right hemicolectomy for a carcinoma of the colon. The caecum had perforated before surgery and the patient has subsequently been septic, requiring inotrope support and ventilation. The consultant has observed that the haemoglobin is 74 g/l and he tells you the patient 'needs a transfusion'.

What do you think?

It has been traditional in intensive care and anaesthetic practice to maintain haemoglobins above 100 g/l, and some have advocated higher goals. The maximisation of oxygen transport in critically ill patients (by optimisation of saturation, haemoglobin and cardiac output), which has had some following over recent years, has led to a trend to maintain higher haemoglobins in some centres. However, recent data suggest that there is no evidence to support keeping haemoglobin levels high. There have been studies suggesting that metastasis rates in patients who have peri-operative transfusion are higher (although some large studies dispute this), and this may also influence against transfusion.

MINI-TUTORIAL

The benefit of transfusion to maintain haemoglobin in critical care patients has been investigated in a randomised controlled multi-centre study. In one group, transfusion was given if the haemoglobin concentration dropped below 70 g/l (haemoglobin concentrations were maintained at 70–90 g/l), and in the second group transfusions were given when the haemoglobin concentration fell below 100 g/l (haemoglobin concentrations were maintained at 100 to 120 g/l. Results: overall, 30 day mortality was similar in the two groups (18.7% vs. 23.3%, $P = 0.11$).

A restrictive strategy (transfusing at 70 g/l) of transfusion appeared to be at least as effective as and possibly superior to a liberal transfusion strategy (transfusing at 100 g/l) in critically ill patients. Patients with acute myocardial infarction or unstable angina may be an exception to this generalisation.

Hebert PC, Wells G, Blajchman MA, Marshall J, Martin C, Pagliarello G, Tweeddale M, Schweitzer I, Yetisir E. A multicenter, randomized, controlled clinical trial of transfusion requirements in critical care. *N. Engl. J. Med.* 1999; **340**(6): 409–17.

13.5 You have admitted a 50-year-old patient with diabetic ketoacidosis to intensive care. He has a tender abdomen with guarding and a high white cell count (17 × 10⁹/l). The surgeon says that he feels that this patient has an acute abdomen and merits a laparotomy. The medical registrar says that a neutrophilia and abdominal signs are a well-recognised feature of diabetic ketoacidosis and he fears that the laparotomy is unwarranted.

The haematology results are available:

Hb	132 g/l
WBC	16.1 × 10⁹/l
Platelets	280 × 10⁹/l
Rbc	4.92 × 10¹²/l
HCT	0.39
MCV	79 fl
MCH	26.8 pg
MCHC	340 g/l

Neutrophils	41%
Lymphocytes	9%
Monocytes	2%
Eosinophils	2%
Basophils	0%
Band	30%
Metamyelocytes	12%
Myelocytes	4%
Promyelocytes	0%
Blasts	0%
NRC	0/100 RBC

Film comment: Neutrophilia, left shift and toxic change.

Do the haematology results help you to resolve the situation?
Yes. The picture on the blood film suggests that this patient has
serious infection. In the absence of other sites and in the presence of
abdominal signs it is likely that he has intra-abdominal sepsis and that
this has provoked his ketoacidosis. This man turned out to have
faecal peritonitis.

MINI-TUTORIAL

Neutrophilia occurs frequently in patients in intensive care in the
absence of infection. Corticosteroids, adrenaline, hypoxia or severe
metabolic disturbance can all provoke neutrophil release.
   There are various features of the neutrophils which suggest that infection is present. These include:

- Granulation – an increase in the staining density and possibly in the number of granules is regularly seen in association with infection (this is generally referred to as 'toxic change').
- Vacuolation – vacuoles in freshly examined neutrophils are usually a sign of severe sepsis.
- Left shift – an increase in less mature neutrophils with less segmentation of their neutrophils is termed 'left shift' and is commonly observed in association with sepsis.
- Band forms – up to 8% of circulating neutrophils are unsegmented, 'band' forms. This percentage increases in sepsis.
- Metamyelocytes and occasional myelocytes are frequently observed in sepsis.
- Observation of the blood film can give a very strong indication that a patient is septic; conversely, an unremarkable film in a patient who has a neutrophilia suggests that the neutrophilia is due to causes other than sepsis (intravenous steroid, adrenaline, a bout of hypoxia, etc.). The blood film is therefore an important investigation in sick patients.

14

X-ray interpretation

14.1 You are asked to check a chest X-ray by one of your colleagues who has inserted a central venous line in a ventilated patient in the ICU (Fig. 14.1).

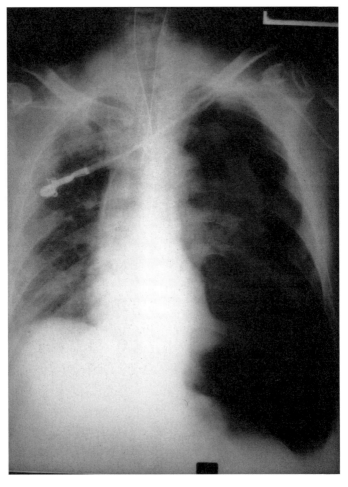

Fig 14.1

What do you think?
There is a left-sided tension pneumothorax (mediastinal displacement, tracheal displacement, diaphragm pushed down). This patient needs an urgent left-sided intercostal catheter.

The central line is in satisfactory position; also noted are ECG electrodes, a radio-opaque nasogastric tube and sternal wires.

14.2 You are urgently asked to come to see a 45-year-old man who is being ventilated following a head injury. He has become hypotensive and tachypnoeic and an urgent chest X-ray has been performed (Fig. 14.2).

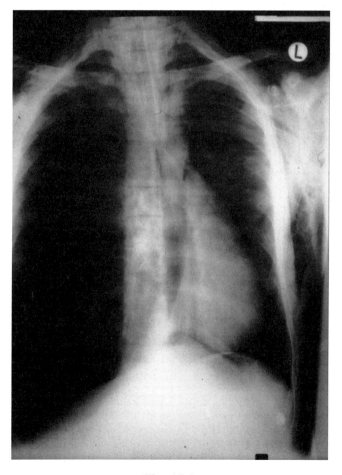

Fig. 14.2

What does the X-ray show?

There is a right-sided tension pneumothorax, with surgical emphysema most evident on the left. The endotracheal tube is in a satisfactory position.

The heart is displaced to the left (you can see vertebrae without heart in front of them, which is abnormal) and the right diaphragm is pushed down. Tension pneumothorax can occur very quickly in ventilated patients. You must be able to diagnose it reliably and rapidly. You must also be confident that you can safely insert an intercostal catheter before taking responsibility for critically ill ventilated patients.

MINI-TUTORIAL

The diaphragm normally forms an acute angle with the chest wall. As pressure increases in the pleural space as a result of pneumothorax the angle becomes rounded. When pressure is high the diaphragm eventually becomes inverted (Fig. 14.3).

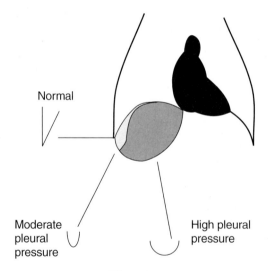

Normal

Moderate pleural pressure

High pleural pressure

Fig. 14.3

Remember that the diaphragm is flimsy and easy to displace. If the mediastinum is shifted away, *but* the angle with the diaphragm is still acute, then it is much more likely that collapse of the other lung is the cause of the mediastinal displacement.

14.3 A 5-year-old child is admitted to the ICU for observation after chest trauma. An intercostal catheter (ICC) has been inserted in the emergency department by the surgical consultant. The child still appears dyspnoeic and is requiring 80% oxygen to maintain arterial oxygen saturations above 90%. An X-ray to check the tube position has been performed (Fig. 14.4).

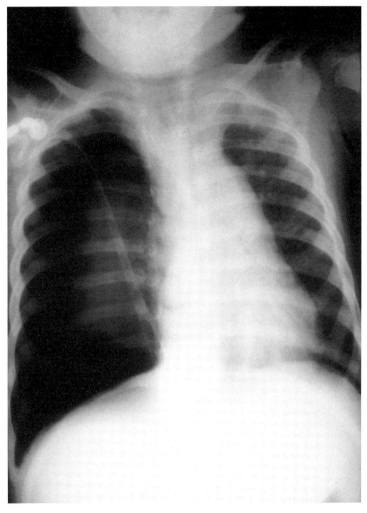

Fig. 14.4

What comments will you make?

The lung remains unexpanded and there are still signs of tension with cardiac and diaphragmatic displacement. The intercostal catheter tip is not in the pleural space (Fig. 14.5).

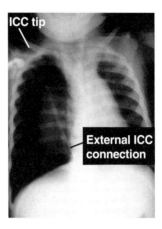

Fig. 14.5

14.4 You review the routine X-ray (Fig. 14.6) of a 16-year-old girl who has severe acute respiratory distress syndrome (ARDS). She is ventilated and has had a chest drain inserted several days earlier because she developed a right-sided pneumothorax. Your colleague, who has just finished the night shift, comments that the right lower zone looks much clearer, which he thinks 'doesn't really fit with the patient', since the oxygenation has deteriorated and inotropes have had to be restarted.

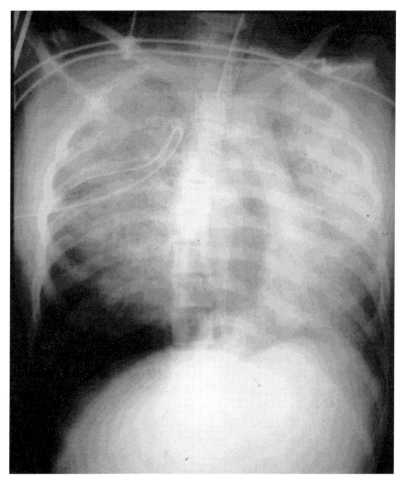

Fig. 14.6

What do you think on review of the X-ray?
There is diffuse pulmonary opacity throughout both lung fields with marked lucency at the right base. The heart is grossly displaced to the left and the right diaphragm is displaced downwards (the angle between the chest wall and diaphragm is not well seen). This girl has a very significant tension pneumothorax which needs urgent drainage. Patients with lung disease or injury can develop loculated pneumothoraces; the presence of a chest drain is no guarantee they do not have tension.

MINI-TUTORIAL

Where the lung is stiff and non-compliant (as in diffuse ARDS) the development of pressure in the pleural space will not squash the lung (which is stiff and resists squashing), so the pressure will squash other more compliant structures in the thorax, the major veins and the heart. Haemodynamic effects may therefore be prominent in the face of what appears to be a small pneumothorax.

14.5 The X-ray of Fig. 14.7 was taken on a Sunday morning following central line insertion. The patient is a 27-year-old motorcyclist who sustained chest and head injuries in an accident. Overnight he was uncooperative and pulled out his arterial line, nasogastric tube and central venous line. All have now been replaced.

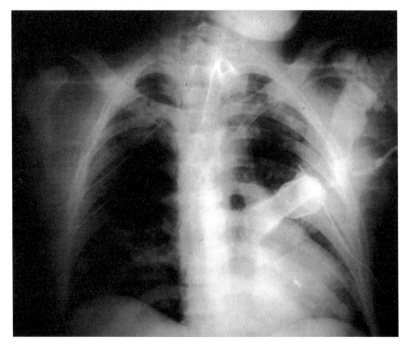

Fig. 14.7

You are asked to look at the film to check the position of the central line.

What do you think?
The left-sided central line is in good position (just below the aortic knuckle, not in the atrium where it may encourage atrial arrhythmias or cause cardiac tamponade if it perforates; see Fig. 14.8). There is no pneumothorax.

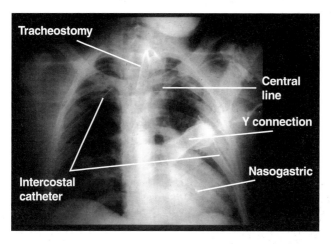

Fig. 14.8

Beware looking at X-rays with only one thing in mind – be thorough. In this case the radio-opaque nasogastric tip is seen behind the heart in the left main bronchus.

The tracheostomy tube and bilateral intercostal tubes should also have been noted.

MINI-TUTORIAL

The structure adjacent to the aortic knuckle on the left in Fig. 14.8 is outside the patient. It is the 'Y' connection of the ventilator circuit.

If you are in doubt about whether something is outside the patient, look at the patient and you will usually easily recognise what it is that you are looking at on the X-ray.

14.6 You are paged to see a 73-year-old woman who had a laparotomy and massive ovarian cyst removed three days earlier. She is generally frail and has been in high dependency since her operation, with difficulty coughing and a requirement for supplemental oxygen (40%).

She has become generally less responsive, with very poor oxygen saturation over the last hour. She is sweating and bradycardic. The X-ray which you requested urgently is available (Fig. 14.9).

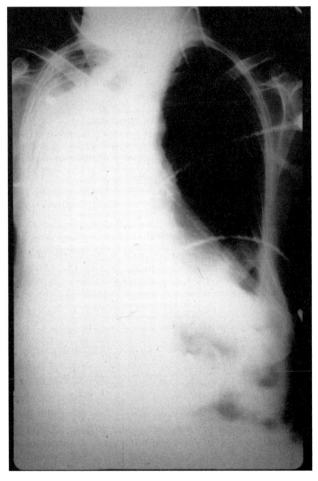

Fig. 14.9

(a) What do you think is going on in the chest?

The right side of the chest is 'whited out'. The trachea is deviated towards the right side, indicating massive collapse of the right lung. In this setting the most likely aetiology is sputum plugging (obstructing tumour or inhaled foreign body are much less likely).

NB: The line running to the left of the heart is external. It is the tube going to the oxygen mask.

(b) What do you think needs to be done?

She is seriously unwell. It is unlikely that physiotherapy will dislodge the plug, and the process may cause her to arrest. She needs intubation with manual hyperinflation (and bronchoscopy if this fails) to move the plug and reinflate the lung.

MINI-TUTORIAL

In cases of massive 'white-out' of a hemithorax the position of the mediastinum (trachea and heart) is important. In massive collapse the mediastinum moves towards the side of the 'white-out', whereas in massive effusion it moves away and with the rare massive consolidation the mediastinum remains in the midline (in consolidation, air broncho-grams are usually evident).

14.7 Following emergency intubation and bagging in this lady, the oxygen saturation (measured by pulse oximetry) improves nicely but then declines again. Following the intubation another X-ray has been taken, which is now back for you to look at (Fig. 14.10).

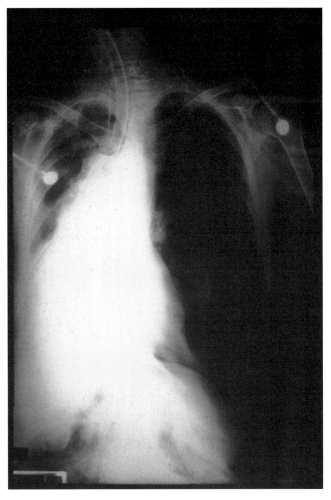

Fig. 14.10

What do you think now?
There is more air in the right lung, but the heart is more displaced to the right. The lower extent of the left diaphragm looks to be below the lower limit of the X-ray (very grossly depressed), and a faint lung edge is visible in the left thorax, so she now has a left tension pneumothorax. She was very frail and multiple lower rib fractures were evident on later review of her films (maybe from coughing, or possibly from physiotherapy or the surgeon). Always expect tension pneumothorax after intubation in a patient with rib fractures.

14.8 A 69-year-old man returned to the general ward after a left pneumonectomy. He has an intercostal catheter *in situ* which is connected to an underwater seal drain. Analgesia with a thoracic epidural was good. On admission he was noted to have some surgical emphysema over the left side of his chest (Fig. 14.11(a)).

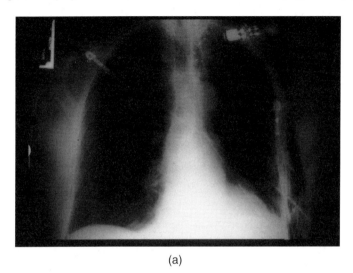

(a)

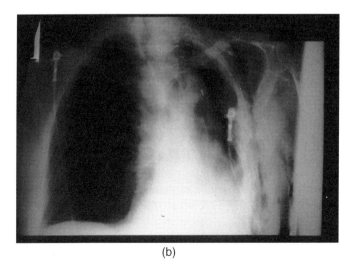

(b)

Fig. 14.11 (a) On admission to ICU; (b) 4 hours after admission to ICU.

Four hours after admission you are urgently called to see the patient because he has suddenly become sweaty, dyspnoeic, tachycardic and hypotensive. An urgent chest X-ray has been taken and is available (Fig. 14.11(b)). The ward nurse is very concerned that he is going to die. She urgently asks you what you want to do.

What will you say?
On the second X-ray (in contrast to the first post-operative X-ray) there is significant loss of volume in the left hemi-thorax with deviation of the trachea and heart (mediastinum) towards the left side.

The underwater drainage is a mistake. The drain should be lifted above the water to permit air to re-enter the left chest. The mediastinum will revert to the midline and the patient will be much improved.

MINI-TUTORIAL

Following pneumonectomy it is important to ensure that there is no midline shift in the immediate post-operative period.

Gradually (over months) the cavity left after the pneumonectomy is reabsorbed and there is eventually marked mediastinal shift; however, this is poorly tolerated when shift occurs rapidly.

If an intercostal catheter is inserted after pneumonectomy it should be clamped. It should *never* be on underwater drain.

Following lobectomy or wedge resection the situation is different, since rapid removal of pleural air and expansion of the remaining lung is important. Underwater drainage is routine following these operations.

14.9 You are asked to review a 34-year-old man who was admitted for observation to the surgical ward overnight having been hit in the stomach by a log in a saw-mill. The surgeons say that he had an unremarkable CT of his abdomen last night and now has no clinical signs of an acute abdomen. He is becoming increasingly dyspnoeic and distressed. His arterial oxygen saturation is poor on high-flow oxygen mask. A chest X-ray has been performed (Fig. 14.12).

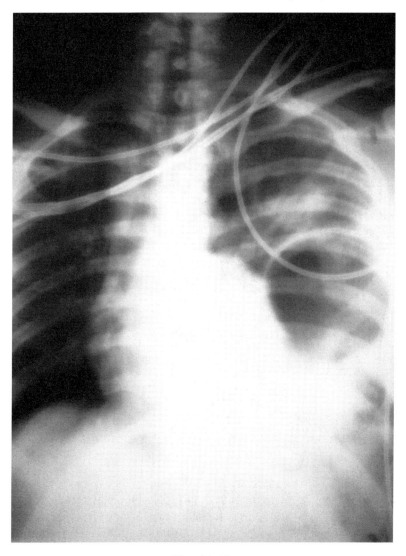

Fig. 14.12

What do you think might be the cause of his respiratory problems?
The stomach is in the left chest. This is the appearance of a ruptured diaphragm.

MINI-TUTORIAL

Diaphragmatic rupture occurs more commonly on the left. Following the tear the negative intra-pleural pressure occurring during respiration tends to progressively suck the fundus of the stomach (or less frequently the colon or spleen) into the chest. As more and more abdominal contents move to the chest respiration may become impeded. The situation may acutely deteriorate if the intra-thoracic bowel becomes obstructed and dilates. In patients who are significantly compromised, paralysis and positive pressure ventilation may provoke acute decompensation.

14.10 Some medical students arrive in ICU with some CT head pictures (Figs 14.13 and 14.14), which they have obtained from the X-ray library. They have come up to ICU because they think that the ICU doctors might be good at explaining the pictures to them. They find you in the tea room.

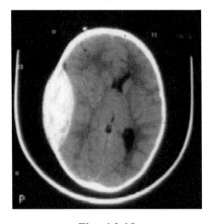 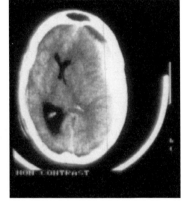

Fig. 14.13   Fig. 14.14

Can you explain the appearances to them?

Fig. 14.13 shows the classic 'lens'-shaped appearance of an extradural haematoma. There is marked ventricular compression and midline shift. Extradural haematomas result from arterial bleeding (often in association with skull fracture), and there is often little underlying brain injury. The patient classically talks after the injury and then becomes increasingly unconscious and dilates a pupil. This is a neurosurgical emergency and with expeditious drainage full recovery can be anticipated.

Fig. 14.14 shows the classic 'new moon' shaped appearance of a subdural haematoma. The inner margin of the haematoma is indistinct as it invaginates into sulci. There is marked ventricular compression and midline shift.

MINI-TUTORIAL

Subdural haematomas result from venous bleeding. In the elderly there is characteristically a history of minimal trauma. Onset is slow with progressive deterioration and recovery can be anticipated following drainage. In younger patients with major neuro-trauma subdural haematomas may occur in association with severe brain shear injury (suggested by loss of grey–white interphase, compression of intracranial CSF and widespread small intracerebral haemorrhages). In such cases little improvement can be anticipated from drainage of the haematoma.

14.11 You are asked to review a 39-year-old man in the Emergency department to consider ICU admission. He presented with a severe sore throat, dysphagia and variable stridor. A lateral neck X-ray has been performed (Fig. 14.15), which the Emergency department resident tells you does not show significant airway obstruction.

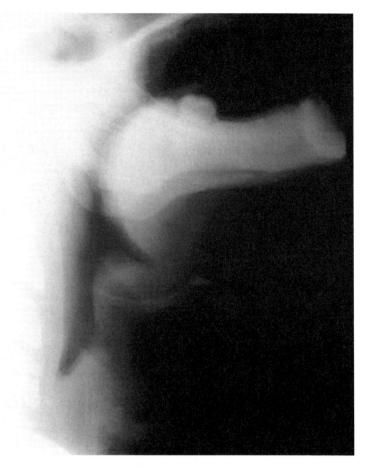

Fig. 14.15

What do you think?
The X-ray shows the classical appearance of epiglottitis. The epiglottis is enlarged and globular on the X-ray (described as being like a 'thumb-print'); see Fig. 14.16(a). Contrast the appearance with the normal epiglottis in Fig. 14.16(b). The retropharyngeal tissues are also thickened (normally the distance from the front of the vertebral column to the airway is not more than 3 mm).

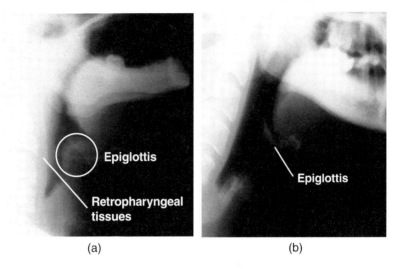

(a)   (b)

Fig. 14.16

MINI-TUTORIAL

Epiglottitis is classically caused by *Haemophillus influenzae* type B (HIB). It previously occurred most frequently in children (with a peak between 2 and 3 years of age), but following the introduction of vaccination has become very infrequent in this group.

Adults now represent the predominant group. In adults there is a wider range of organisms causing the clinical picture and the symptoms and signs may be less clear than in children.

Dixon J, Black JJ. Adult supraglottitis: an important cause of airway obstruction. *J. Accid. Emerg. Med.* 1998; **15**(2): 114–15.

15

Trauma

15.1 You are involved in the initial resuscitation of a 45-year-old man who has suffered a traumatic amputation of his right leg. On arrival in the Emergency department he has a blood pressure of 50/30 and a pulse rate of 126/minute. The ambulance officers have failed to find a vein and have rapidly transported him. An intravenous cannula is now in place.
   The registrar asks you to get some intravenous fluid.

What will you bring?
Either crystalloid or colloid are appropriate initial fluids to administer. More crystalloid will be required to obtain the same effect. There is likely to have been significant blood loss and consideration of early blood transfusion is appropriate.

MINI-TUTORIAL

The two major fluid types which are used for resuscitation are crystalloid solutions (e.g. normal saline or Hartmann's solution) and colloid solutions (e.g. albumin or Haemaccel).
   Colloids exert colloid osmotic pressure while crystalloids do not.
   The initial intravascular volume expansion is less when crystalloids are used (2–3 times the volume of crystalloid is required to achieve the same end point; e.g. blood pressure or CVP). Consequently, more weight gain and tissue oedema results following crystalloid-based resuscitation.
   The use of hypertonic saline solutions (e.g. 7.5% saline) or mixtures of colloid and hypertonic saline are gaining favour for the initial resuscitation of trauma. In this situation the intravascular expansion is much greater than the infused volume and resuscitation goals are achieved with small volumes of intravenous infusion (and are therefore more likely to be achieved and achieved quickly). This form of resuscitation may be particularly useful in head-injured patients where rapid restoration of blood pressure coupled with a reduction in cerebral oedema is likely to be associated with improved outcome.
   Glucose solutions are not appropriate for resuscitation, since they rapidly distribute to the intra-cellular space (and consequently there is minimal intravascular volume expansion).

Simma B, Burger R, Falk M, Sacher P, Fanconi S. A prospective, randomized, and controlled study of fluid management in children with severe head injury: lactated Ringer's solution versus hypertonic saline. *Crit. Care Med.* 1998; **26**(7): 1265–70.

A rough approximation of the intravascular volume increment following infusion of the various fluid types can be derived by considering the relative volumes of the different spaces: total body fluid (40 litres), extra-cellular fluid (12 litres), intravascular fluid/plasma volume (3 litres).

1000 ml 5% glucose distributes throughout the total body fluid (40 litres).

Thus 3/40 of this will be in the intravascular space = 75 ml intravascular expansion per litre infused.

1000 ml N/saline distributes throughout extra-cellular fluid (12 litres).

3/12 or 1/4 will be in the intravascular space = 250 ml intravascular expansion per litre infused.

1000 ml plasma (or blood) distributes throughout the intravascular space only (at least immediately after infusion).

All will be in the intravascular space = 1000 ml intravascular expansion per litre infused.

15.2   You have admitted a 23-year-old man with a head injury to the Intensive Care Unit. He has had a CT scan which shows some frontal contusion and diffuse cerebral oedema. He has a Glasgow Coma Score of 8 and is intubated.
    The surgical registrar loudly asserts that evidence does not support the routine use of hyperventilation in head injury. A medical student attached to the ICU asks about this, as he has previously heard that both mannitol or hyperventilation are effective.

What will you tell him?
The registrar is right. Routine hyperventilation is contraindicated and it is recommended that a $P_a\text{CO}_2$ of < 35 mmHg (4.66 kPa) is avoided during the first 24 hours after severe head injury.

MINI-TUTORIAL

Raised intracranial pressure can be rapidly reduced by acute hyperventilation, and this treatment been used routinely over the last 20 years.

It is clear that cerebral blood flow following severe head injury is less than half of that in normal individuals, and that this falls further in the face of hyperventilation, with an increased risk of causing cerebral ischaemia.

Recent clinical studies have failed to show benefit, and on the contrary have been associated with adverse outcomes.

Brief periods of hyperventilation may be necessary for acute neurological deterioration refractory to other treatment, but close monitoring for cerebral hypoxia is recommended when hyperventilation is employed.

The use of hyperventilation in the management of severe traumatic brain injury. *J. Neurotrauma* 1996; **13**: 699–703.

15.3 A 25-year-old man is brought in to hospital after falling from the top of a hay shed. He is conscious but complains that his chest is painful and he is having difficulty breathing. He obviously has a fracture of his left femur and both tibias.

An iv is *in situ* and he has been given 500 ml Haemaccel and 500 ml N/saline on his way to hospital. He has an oxygen mask on at 15 l/min flow.

On examination he has a flail segment right chest with reduced breath sounds on the right. His heart rate is 140/min, BP 150/80, and respiratory rate 42/min.

The pulse oximetry is not reading well, but intermittently there is a reading of 80% S_pO_2.

Arrangements have been made for him to be admitted to another hospital (because your hospital is on by-pass). The ambulance is ready to take the patient and the ambulance officers are keen to do so.

Do you feel he is fit to transfer?
No, he is certainly not fit to transfer.

This is an important issue, which is often delegated to inexperienced staff. Perceived urgency often prevents considered thought.

Readiness to transfer needs to be considered in basic terms – airway, breathing, circulation.

His airway is satisfactory.

Breathing is unstable. He is hyperventilating. This may be due to thoracic problems or he may be hyperventilating to compensate for metabolic acidosis. In either case he is not stable.

He is also hypoxic (S_pO_2 80%). This is probably due to thoracic injury which requires investigation. He may require intubation and ventilation. An intercostal catheter may be indicated.

Circulation is unstable. He is inadequately resuscitated. His pulse rate is too high. Although the blood pressure is normal, this is not the most sensitive indicator of hypovolaemia. Where practical, demonstration of a postural drop is suggestive of hypovolaemia.

Poor peripheral perfusion is a common cause of failure of the pulse oximeter to function reliably.

He has fractures which can predictably be associated with at least 4 unit blood loss.

Thirst, urine output and low JVP may be other indicators of hypovolaemia. His fractures have not been stabilised. Stabilisation is likely to reduce further blood loss, reduce the chance of fat embolism syndrome and minimise pain during transfer.

15.4 You are asked to transfer a 56-year-old lady to the CT scanner. She is ventilated on a transport mechanical ventilator for the trip at 600 ml tidal volume and at a rate of 16 breaths per minute on 100% oxygen. You have a C size cylinder and the gauge on the cylinder indicates that it is two thirds full.

How long is the oxygen likely to last?
She is using 9.6 litres of oxygen per minute (600 ml × 16). A full size C contains 490 litres, so there will be about 330 litres in a cylinder which is two thirds full. This will last about 30 minutes.

MINI-TUTORIAL

It is useful to know the capacity of cylinders, particularly of the smaller cylinders:

C cylinder	490 litres	E cylinder	4100 litres
D cylinder	1630 litres	G cylinder	8280 litres

It is important to start with a full cylinder, to take spares where there is any suggestion that they may run out, only to change from wall oxygen just prior to departure and to re-use oxygen from the wall or larger cylinders as soon as possible.

It is important to be aware that some transport ventilators are designed to have a continuous leak of about 1 l/min and this should be taken into consideration. Of more significance is the *very rapid use of oxygen when venturi suction is used.*

Most transport ventilators will only operate when there is a source of compressed oxygen. If the oxygen runs out the ventilator will not function. It is essential to carry a manual bag-and-mask whenever you transport a patient from the ICU.

15.5 You are instructed to maintain the cerebral perfusion pressure of a patient who has had a head injury at greater than 70 mmHg. He currently has a mean blood pressure of 80 mmHg.

Are you happy that his cerebral perfusion pressure (CPP) is > 70 mmHg?

No. The CPP is the mean arterial pressure minus the intra-cranial pressure. Consequently you must know the intra-cranial pressure (ICP) to derive the CPP.

MINI-TUTORIAL

Whether the use of intra-cranial pressure (ICP) monitoring results in improved outcome after severe head injury has not been demonstrated by prospective, randomized clinical trial. However, most neurosurgical centres have come to rely on data from ICP monitoring to direct management. Consequently a placebo-controlled trial of ICP monitoring would now probably be impossible.

Monitoring of intra-cerebral pressure helps to predict cerebral herniation and permits calculation of the cerebral perfusion pressure. CPP is an important determinant of cerebral blood flow (in the absence of effective auto-regulation) and low CPP is associated with cerebral ischaemia. Maintaining the CPP at above 70 mmHg is a generally accepted goal.

The level of ICP which requires treatment remains a matter of debate. Most clinicians would treat an ICP of 20 mmHg.

15.6 You are asked to help with the management of a 19-year-old male with a severe head injury in the Emergency department. He has a Glasgow Coma Score of 6 and has been intubated and ventilated. A CT scan shows no focal haemorrhage. His pulse rate is 110/minute and blood pressure 90/60. Blood gases show a P_aO_2 of 78 mmHg (10.37 kPa) and a P_aCO_2 of 38 mmHg (5.05 kPa).

His transfer to a regional trauma centre is arranged and a retrieval team are on their way. The Emergency department is very busy and you are asked to help by looking after him for a few minutes.

Is there anything about his current management which requires urgent attention?

A blood pressure of 87/60 is totally unsatisfactory in a patient who has suffered a severe head injury. If there are signs of hypovolaemia then infusion of fluid (crystalloid or colloid) is appropriate; otherwise, starting an infusion of vasoconstrictor (e.g. aramine or noradrenaline) is appropriate.

MINI-TUTORIAL

Secondary brain insults, particularly hypotension (systolic blood pressure < 95 mmHg) and hypoxia (P_aO_2 < 60 mmHg), are the most important determinants of outcome following severe head injury.

In particular, hypotension occurs frequently (in about 33% of severely head injured patients) and is associated with a threefold increase in mortality. Hypotension has been recognised to occur not only during transfer but during care in ICU.

Improved outcomes from head injury can be anticipated if more of those involved in the care of head-injured patients recognise the importance of maintaining the blood pressure, increase monitoring of blood pressure in these patients and initiate simple therapeutic manoeuvres immediately hypotension is detected.

Chesnut RM. Secondary brain insults after head injury: clinical perspectives. *New Horiz.* 1995; **3**(3): 366–75.
Chesnut RM, Marshall LF, Klauber MR, Blunt BA, Baldwin N, Eisenberg HM, Jane JA, Marmarou A, Foulkes MA. The role of secondary brain injury in determining outcome from severe head injury. *J. Trauma* 1993; **34**(2): 216–22.

15.7 A junior doctor from the Emergency department speaks to you about a case with which he was associated. A 38 kg 11-year-old boy presented with an extra-dural haematoma following a head injury. He was unconscious, irritable and extending to pain. He was intubated with a size 5.5 un-cuffed ETT. He was ventilated with a Laerdal bag and was given vecuronium 2 mg iv when he started to 'cough on the tube'.

He was then transported to the regional paediatric neurosurgical centre with the Emergency department doctor. During transport it was noted that he was initially coughing and developed a large leak around his tube.

On arrival at the neurosurgical centre the child was observed to have fixed dilated pupils, was felt to be ventilating poorly and had a $P_a co_2$ of 90 mmHg (12 kPa). Despite urgent neurosurgery he was subsequently certified brain dead.

The junior doctor is naturally upset and is wondering what could have been done better to avoid this awful outcome.

What do you think?

It sounds like this junior and inexperienced doctor managed the boy without supervision. Were senior staff aware? Were they called to assist?

The endotracheal tube size is much too small for the age of the child. There are tables which predict average tube sizes and insertion distances for various ages. Doctors who infrequently manage children should refer to these tables.

Was it appropriate to transfer him or could emergency surgery have been done locally? Was there consultation and discussion about this at a senior level? Often these discussions occur at junior level and all options are not considered and discussed.

Vecuronium has a predictable action for 20–30 minutes so it should have been anticipated that the effect would wear off during transport, with a predictable increase in the leak. Provision to maintain the block would have been appropriate

It is important to match the experience/expertise of the escorting staff to the needs and anticipated problems associated with the transfer.

16

General management issues

16.1 A doctor who has just been rostered to ICU asks you about APACHE.

What is APACHE?
APACHE stands for Acute Physiology And Chronic Heath Evaluation. It is a measure of severity of illness on ICU admission.

MINI-TUTORIAL

APACHE II has 12 physiological variables and weightings for the presence of one of several defined chronic illnesses, for the urgency of admission (elective vs. emergency) and for age. The worst physiological results occurring during the first 24 hours of ICU admission are recorded.

Glasgow Coma Score should not reflect the effect of sedation; presedation scores should be used. Scoring sedated patients is a mistaken way to get big APACHE scores. A recent survey has revealed very poor consistency about the way that the Glasgow Coma Score is assigned to ventilated patients. Since the Glasgow Coma Score constitutes up to 12 points in the APACHE score this can have an enormous effect on the overall score. Great caution should be exercised when one unit is compared with another until improved consistency of scoring is achieved.

By associating APACHE scores with a diagnostic category a risk of death can be calculated. When these are added together for a number of admissions this can be compared with actual hospital mortality to give an index of unit performance. The prediction of mortality for individual patients is not strong enough for any clinical decision making to be based on this.

While APACHE II is most widely used there is now an APACHE III. This has 17 variables and an assessment of immune status. The predictions are somewhat more accurate, but the algorithms are commercial (APACHE II is public) and expensive.

There are other similar severity of illness scoring systems (e.g. SAPS: Simplified Acute Physiology Score) which have enjoyed less widespread application than APACHE.

Buechler CM, Blostein PA, Koestner A, Hurt K, Schaars M, McKernan J. Variation among trauma centers' calculation of Glasgow Coma Scale score: results of a national survey. *J. Trauma* 1998; **45**(3): 429–32.

Knaus WA, Draper EA, Wagner DP and Zimmerman JE. APACHE II: a severity of disease classification system. *Crit. Care Med.* 1985; **10**: 818–29.

16.2 At 1 a.m. you are shown some arterial blood gases from a 65-year-old man who is on the medical ward. He has a diagnosis of lobar pneumonia and was admitted at 8 p.m. At the time of admission he had arterial blood gases measured, which were as follows:

P_aO_2	34 mmHg	(4.52 kPa)
P_aCO_2	27 mmHg	(3.59 kPa)
BIC	20 mmol/l	

At the time he was prescribed 50% oxygen, cefotaxime 2 g 12 hourly and physiotherapy.
The 1 a.m. gases are as follows:

P_aO_2	32 mmHg	(4.26 kPa)
P_aCO_2	49 mmHg	(6.52 kPa)
BIC	15 mmol/l	

The resident who has done the gases asks your advice.

What will you say?
The additional oxygen has had no effect (probably because the patient has deteriorated over the last few hours). The patient certainly needs more oxygen (a P_aO_2 of 32 mmHg/4.26 kPa is dangerously low) and monitoring to observe whether the saturation or P_aO_2 improve. Should rapid improvement not occur, intubation and mechanical ventilation are urgently required.

Additionally the bicarbonate has fallen and the CO_2 has risen, indicating increasing metabolic acidosis and reduced respiratory compensation, both of which suggest progressive deterioration and are worrying.

It is likely that no antibiotic has been administered (see below), and this should be checked.

MINI-TUTORIAL

It is vital in sick patients to check that important antibiotics have been administered. Writing a 12 hourly dose at 8 p.m. when drugs are given at 6 a.m. and 6 p.m. is likely to result in no dose being given for 10 hours after prescription (unless nursing staff are alert and suggest an additional dose). On starting important drugs such as antibiotics in sick patients you should write a 'stat' dose to ensure a dose is given immediately.

16.3 While in the residents' quarters you hear about a sick 70-year-old with pneumonia and shock. The medical registrar assures you that she 'is not an ICU candidate', having had a dense hemiplegia 6 months before and subsequent poor health. Four hours later a code is called when this lady suffers a cardio-pulmonary arrest. She cannot be extubated after resuscitation and an ICU bed is requested by the medical team.

The medical intern is apologetic and suggests that things have been 'a bit messed up'. He wonders what might have been done to avoid this situation.

Do you have any suggestions?
It is very important to have a clear agreed plan of management. If a limited treatment strategy is selected then it is more likely that the patient will deteriorate than where intensive treatment is instituted. When such a patient arrests it is illogical to suddenly change tack and institute full resuscitation and ICU support. In general, where less than fully committed management on the ward is considered appropriate the role of cardiopulmonary resuscitation should be seriously considered. In most cases it will not be rational, and discussions with the patient, family and senior medical staff should be initiated (often with your urging).

In summary: do not leave patients with instruction for limited treatment without consideration of their CPR status (and don't let others do it).

16.4 An 83-year-old man is admitted to ICU having become shocked during a TURP. This is thought to be a result of bacteraemia from prostatitis. He had metaraminol and adrenaline (20 ml 1:10 000) in theatre and is still on an adrenaline infusion (0.4 μg/kg/min) and remains intubated.

As a consequence of his incomplete resection there is marked post-operative bleeding (the catheter drainage looks like frank blood).

The urologist states that he feels the patient is 'a bit of a poor old thing' and says that he 'only thinks it is worth giving him 4 units of blood'.

When you report the admission to the ICU specialist he asks if you are comfortable about the management plan.

Are you?

No. Limitation of treatment is common and often appropriate, but it is essentially based on an agreement between the patient, their relatives, the doctors and nursing staff. Where any of these disagree there will be stress and the potential for significant dispute. When these decisions are made you must confirm that communication has occurred and there is agreement. This can be time-consuming, particularly when you are busy, but failure can get you into lots of trouble.

In this case the family were called after the 4 units of blood were given and continuing blood loss caused ongoing hypovolaemic shock. His son was very angry that his father was not being resuscitated and stated that his father was fit and well yesterday (the patient's wife felt just the same). He demanded that the urologist be called, and the patient was resuscitated and internal iliac arteries were ligated, which controlled the bleeding. As a consequence of the prolonged shock before reinstitution of resuscitation the man was left in a vegetative state. Significant money changed hands as a consequence of the mismanagement of the case.

16.5 A new intern who is covering the surgical wards overnight asks your advice. She has been seeing a 63-year-old man who has had haematemesis and melaena following an ERCP and sphincterotomy. He has a history of hypertension (160/100) but was on no treatment.

He has just opened his bowels again and has passed frank blood and clots.

The intern says he is 'a bit clammy' and has become hypotensive (80/60). She has rung the surgical registrar, who has suggested continued close observation.

A drip is in progress and 1000 ml 5% glucose has been ordered over 12 hours.

The intern asks if there is anything else she should be doing.

What will you say?

What is the haemoglobin? Is his coagulation normal? Is he passing urine?

Blood loss sufficient to cause *both* haematemesis and melaena is always of reasonable volume. If the source is upper GI and frank blood is lost from the rectum (rather than melaena) then the bleeding is very significant.

Hypotension in response to haemorrhage indicates that the compensation is failing. This is serious, particularly if the patient has signs of poor perfusion (cold, clammy periphery).

This man needs intravascular volume urgently. To drop his blood pressure to this extent the patient has lost at least 1000 ml of blood. Replacement needs to be fast. Blood, colloid or crystalloid are indicated. 5% glucose is not appropriate since it has a wider volume of distribution (see 15.1).

Management of this patient needs to be based on some goals (such as restoring the systolic blood pressure to 130 or getting a urine output of 30 ml/h). The intravenous fluid needs to be given quickly to try to attain these goals. If bleeding continues and the goals are not achieved with rapid transfusion then the surgeon needs to be called again. Failure to have goals, or to communicate them, often leads to prolonged periods of inadequate care.

The surgical registrar may require some re-education.

Although this scenario revolves around hypotension a similar process of goal setting and review is important when managing hypoxia, oliguria, etc.

16.6 At 3 a.m. you are asked to urgently review a 74-year-old man who was admitted to ICU following injection of oesophageal varices the day before. He has had a large haematemesis and is now shocked (BP 60/45, pulse 140/min, clammy periphery, tachypnoeic, cyanotic). You ring the registrar who suggests giving him 'some Haemaccel' and 'keeping a close eye on him'. He then puts down the phone.

You (I hope) are not convinced this is appropriate management.

What should you have done differently to achieve a better outcome?

Try to think what needs to be done for the patient before you phone. Then you can raise this before the phone call comes to an end. Try to be very clear in your own mind when you are calling for help.

If you want someone to come then be sure to clearly say so – 'I think you need to see him', 'I'm very worried about him, I think he is going to die. It might be good if you were to have seen him' – or something similar works wonders (you will notice good nursing staff do the same to you!). Insist nicely: it is inevitable that when they see the patient they will change their tune about the wisdom of seeing your moribund patient.

In addition, try to think what questions will be asked and have answers ready. You will present yourself as an idiot if you rush from the phone to get information every time a question is asked.

Good luck and enjoy your ICU rotation!

Index